PHYSICAL FITNESS AND EXERCISE

AN OVERVIEW

PHYSICAL FITNESS, DIET AND EXERCISE

Additional books and e-books in this series can be found on Nova's website under the Series tab.

PHYSICAL FITNESS, DIET AND EXERCISE

PHYSICAL FITNESS AND EXERCISE

AN OVERVIEW

QUINZIA TREVISANO
EDITOR

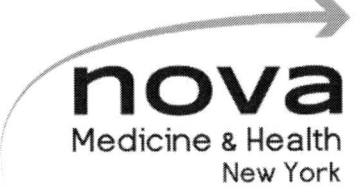

Copyright © 2020 by Nova Science Publishers, Inc.

All rights reserved. No part of this book may be reproduced, stored in a retrieval system or transmitted in any form or by any means: electronic, electrostatic, magnetic, tape, mechanical photocopying, recording or otherwise without the written permission of the Publisher.

We have partnered with Copyright Clearance Center to make it easy for you to obtain permissions to reuse content from this publication. Simply navigate to this publication's page on Nova's website and locate the "Get Permission" button below the title description. This button is linked directly to the title's permission page on copyright.com. Alternatively, you can visit copyright.com and search by title, ISBN, or ISSN.

For further questions about using the service on copyright.com, please contact:
Copyright Clearance Center
Phone: +1-(978) 750-8400   Fax: +1-(978) 750-4470   E-mail: info@copyright.com.

NOTICE TO THE READER

The Publisher has taken reasonable care in the preparation of this book, but makes no expressed or implied warranty of any kind and assumes no responsibility for any errors or omissions. No liability is assumed for incidental or consequential damages in connection with or arising out of information contained in this book. The Publisher shall not be liable for any special, consequential, or exemplary damages resulting, in whole or in part, from the readers' use of, or reliance upon, this material. Any parts of this book based on government reports are so indicated and copyright is claimed for those parts to the extent applicable to compilations of such works.

Independent verification should be sought for any data, advice or recommendations contained in this book. In addition, no responsibility is assumed by the Publisher for any injury and/or damage to persons or property arising from any methods, products, instructions, ideas or otherwise contained in this publication.

This publication is designed to provide accurate and authoritative information with regard to the subject matter covered herein. It is sold with the clear understanding that the Publisher is not engaged in rendering legal or any other professional services. If legal or any other expert assistance is required, the services of a competent person should be sought. FROM A DECLARATION OF PARTICIPANTS JOINTLY ADOPTED BY A COMMITTEE OF THE AMERICAN BAR ASSOCIATION AND A COMMITTEE OF PUBLISHERS.

Additional color graphics may be available in the e-book version of this book.

Library of Congress Cataloging-in-Publication Data

Names: Trevisano, Quinzia, editor. Title: Physical fitness and exercise : an overview / Quinzia Trevisano.
Description: New York : Nova Science Publishers, [2020] | Series: Physical fitness, diet and exercise | Includes bibliographical references and index. | Summary: "This compilation discusses how low levels of physical activity and excess body weight are considered key health risks in modern societies. This may be attributed to changes in the social and built environment, along with technical advances that reduced the requirement for physical activity in daily living. The authors investigate population aging, the physiology of aging, and the prescription of physical activity for the elderly. In addition, the effects of oxidative stress on skeletal muscle during high-intense resistance training are studied, particularly focusing on reactive oxygen species"-- Provided by publisher.
Identifiers: LCCN 2020038891 (print) | LCCN 2020038892 (ebook) | ISBN 9781536185218 (paperback) | ISBN 9781536185959 (adobe pdf) Subjects: LCSH: Exercise--Health aspects. | Physical fitness--Health aspects. | Exercise--Physiological aspects. | Physical fitness--Physiological aspects. | Physical fitness for older people.
Classification: LCC RA781 .P5649 2020 (print) | LCC RA781 (ebook) | DDC 613.7--dc23
LC record available at https://lccn.loc.gov/2020038891
LC ebook record available at https://lccn.loc.gov/2020038892

Published by Nova Science Publishers, Inc. † New York

Contents

Preface		vii
Chapter 1	Associations of Physical Activity, Physical Fitness and Body Weight: Implications for Weight Management *Clemens Drenowatz and Klaus Greier*	1
Chapter 2	Aging Physiology and Physical Activity Prescription for Elderly *Eduardo Borba Neves,* *Gabrielle Cristine Moura Fernandes Pucci* *and Francisco Jose Félix Saavedra*	35
Chapter 3	Effects of High-Intensity Resistance Training on Oxidative Stress *Eduardo Borba Neves, Danielli Braga de Mello,* *Rogério Santos de Aguiar,* *Juliana Brandão Pinto de Castro* *and Rodrigo Gomes de Souza Vale*	71
Index		139

PREFACE

This compilation discusses how low levels of physical activity and excess body weight are considered key health risks in modern societies. This may be attributed to changes in the social and built environment, along with technical advances that reduced the requirement for physical activity in daily living. The authors investigate population aging, the physiology of aging, and the prescription of physical activity for the elderly. In addition, the effects of oxidative stress on skeletal muscle during high-intense resistance training are studied, particularly focusing on reactive oxygen species.

Chapter 1 - Low levels of physical activity (PA) and excess body weight are considered key health risks in modern societies. This may, at least partly, be attributed to changes in the social and built environment along with technical advances that reduced the requirement for PA in daily living while sedentary behaviors have become increasingly popular. Along with these developments fitness levels and motor competence have declined as well. Even though considerable efforts have been made to address these problems, overweight/obesity rates continue to increase or have stabilized at high levels and a large amount of people remains insufficiently active. The limited success of current intervention strategies also reflects a lack of understanding of the regulation of body weight and the reciprocal association with PA, physical fitness and motor competence. In fact it can be argued that energy flux (i.e., rate of energy expenditure and energy intake) rather than body weight or energy balance is a regulated. This means that human beings need to achieve a certain level of energy energy expenditure that is matched by a similar energy intake. In case of low PA energy expenditure can be increased by increasing body mass and, therefore, excess weight gain may be a physiologically normal response in conditions of low PA. In order to promote a sufficient amount of PA, physical fitness and motor competence appear to be critical components as they facilitate participation in various forms of PA, including exercise. Accordingly, motor dvelopment and physical fitness should be emphasized at young ages to encourage an active lifestyle beyond childhood and adoelscence.

Chapter 2 - This chapter presents the aging physiology and concepts for physical activity prescription for the elderly. To this end, the following topics will be discussed: population aging and its challenges; stages and types of aging; physiology of aging (anthropometric changes, cardiac system, respiratory system, nervous system, musculoskeletal system, immune system, and endocrine system); prescription of physical activity for the elderly (concept of physical fitness, muscle strength/endurance training, flexibility training, balance training, cardiorespiratory or aerobic training); and some final considerations. Exercises should be aimed at facilitating the daily lives of the elderly, aiming to work on the needed physical skills for maintaining the autonomy and independence of this population. In this sense, functional activities should be prioritized, thinking about the basic movements that the elderly perform most in their daily lives, such as, for example, walking, getting up from a chair, showering, getting dressed, putting on a shoe.

Chapter 3 - This chapter presents the effects of Oxidative Stress (OS) in skeletal muscle during high-intense resistance training (HIRT). To this end, the following topics will be discussed: high-intense resistance training, Oxidative stress, effects of high-intensity resistance training in skeletal muscle, definition of oxidative stress and reactive oxygen species (ROS), antioxidant defense system, and some final considerations. HIRT results in oxidative damage to macromolecules in blood and skeletal muscle. During HIRT, the metabolic rate in active skeletal muscle increases more than 100 times when compared to the levels at rest. The associated increase in oxygen consumption raises the ROS-s rate in skeletal muscle that have an impact on reducing muscle strength production. ROS produced during exercise leads to increased expression of endogenous antioxidants. These antioxidant molecules have the function of preventing the negative effects of ROS on the muscles, neutralizing free radicals. Also, ROS seems to be involved in the adaptation induced by the exercise of the muscle phenotype.

In: Physical Fitness and Exercise
Editor: Quinzia Trevisano

ISBN: 978-1-53618-521-8
© 2020 Nova Science Publishers, Inc.

Chapter 1

ASSOCIATIONS OF PHYSICAL ACTIVITY, PHYSICAL FITNESS AND BODY WEIGHT: IMPLICATIONS FOR WEIGHT MANAGEMENT

Clemens Drenowatz[1,] and Klaus Greier[2,3]*

[1]Division of Physical Education,
University of Education Upper Austria, Linz, Austria
[2]Division of Physical Education,
Private University of Education (KPH-ES), Stams, Austria
[3]Departent of Sport Science, University of Innsbruck,
Innsbruck, Austria

ABSTRACT

Low levels of physical activity (PA) and excess body weight are considered key health risks in modern societies. This may, at least partly, be attributed to changes in the social and built environment along with technical advances that reduced the requirement for PA in daily living while sedentary behaviors have become increasingly popular. Along with these developments fitness levels and motor competence have declined as

---

[*] Corresponding Author's E-mail: Clemens.drenowatz@ph-ooe.at.

well. Even though considerable efforts have been made to address these problems, overweight/obesity rates continue to increase or have stabilized at high levels and a large amount of people remains insufficiently active.

The limited success of current intervention strategies also reflects a lack of understanding of the regulation of body weight and the reciprocal association with PA, physical fitness and motor competence. In fact it can be argued that energy flux (i.e., rate of energy expenditure and energy intake) rather than body weight or energy balance is a regulated. This means that human beings need to achieve a certain level of energy energy expenditure that is matched by a similar energy intake. In case of low PA energy expenditure can be increased by increasing body mass and, therefore, excess weight gain may be a physiologically normal response in conditions of low PA. In order to promote a sufficient amount of PA, physical fitness and motor competence appear to be critical components as they facilitate participation in various forms of PA, including exercise. Accordingly, motor dvelopment and physical fitness should be emphasized at young ages to encourage an active lifestyle beyond childhood and adoelscence.

Keywords: health promotion, motor competence, energy flux, energy balance, body weight, overweight, obesity

INTRODUCTION

Insufficient physical activity (PA) has serious implications on a person's health and well-being, including an increased risk for excess body weight, cardiovascular and metabolic diseases, certain types of cancer, depression and all-cause mortality (O'Donovan et al. 2010). Further, expected lifetime without illness is 8-10 years shorter in sedentary compared to physically active people (Brønnum-Hansen et al. 2007). Accordingly, physical inactivity is considered one of the leading causes of disability and death (Kohl et al. 2012). In fact, it is the second highest behavioral risk factor, only superseded by smoking (World Health Organization 2010). Nevertheless, more than 1/3 of adults in high-income countries are considered insufficiently active (Guthold et al. 2018) and only 25% of adolescents (aged 11-17 years) meet current PA recommendations (World Health Organisation 2018). Given the estimated annual costs of 54 billion US dollars in direct health care and 14 billion US dollars associated with lost productivity, which reflect between 1% and 3% of national health care costs, physical inactivity also puts a significant burden on the society (World Health Organisation 2018).

Of particular concern is the increase in the prevalence of physical inactivity despite considerable efforts, especially in high-income countries (Guthold et al. 2018). This may, at least partly, be attributed to changes in the social and built environment. Technical advances contributed to a decline in occupational PA over the last several decades (Church et al. 2011) and reduced the physical demands during household activities (Archer et al. 2013). Sedentary behaviors such as high media consumption, on the other hand, have become increasingly popular and contribute to a sedentary lifestyle (Dollman, Norton, and Norton 2005, Biddle et al. 2017). Low PA levels are further associated with a decline in physical fitness and motor abilities, particularly during childhood and adolescence (Roth et al. 2010, O'Brien, Belton, and Issartel 2016, Tomkinson, Lang, and Tremblay 2019). Accordingly, available data indicates that only 50% of children can be considered competent across a broad range of motor skills (Bryant, Duncan, and Birch 2014, Hardy et al. 2013, Goodway, Robinson, and Crowe 2010). Given the reciprocal interaction between motor competence, physical fitness and PA this may lead to a vicious cycle of low PA, low physical fitness and poor motor competence (Greier and Drenowatz 2018, Stodden et al. 2008). In fact, the lack of success of current PA interventions has, at least partly, been attributed to a lack of consideraton towards physical fitness and motor competence (Cattuzzo et al. 2016, Rodrigues, Stodden, and Lopes 2016).

Another detrimental correlate of insufficient PA and low motor competence is increased body weight (Barnett et al. 2016, Bremer and Cairney 2016). As has been shown for low PA, excess body weight is associated with various detrimental health effects, including cardiovascular and metabolic disease, poor pulmonary function, orthopedic problems, depressive symptoms and overall quality of life (Reilly et al. 2003, Lobstein et al. 2004). The rising prevalence of childhood obesity is of particular concern as it increases the risk for adult obesity (Wang and Lobstein 2006, Finkelstein et al. 2012, Singh et al. 2008). Further, children with excess body weight have an increased risk for metabolic problems at young ages and chronic disease as well as premature death even in the absence of adult obesity (Sinha et al. 2002, Umer et al. 2017).

Even though weight gain is a multifactorial problem, including genes and the environment, the rapid rise in the prevalence of obesity over a relatively short period of time suggests that behavioral choices such as participation in PA along with dietary intake play a critical role in long-term weight management (Hill et al. 2003, Hall 2018). In the United States, for example, obesity rates have tripled in 40 years (Flegal et al. 2010) and the average body weight of children increased by 5 kg over the last 30 years (Lobstein et al. 2015). Nevertheless, there remains controversy on the independent role of PA and exercise in weight management (Dhurandhar et al. 2015, Shaw et al. 2006, Melanson et al. 2013), which may in part be attributed to a limited understanding of the energy balance model.

The research presented in this chapter aims to enhance the understanding of the complex interaction of physical activity, physical fitness, motor competence and body weight. Given the importance of PA in the regulation of energy balance and the fact that PA tracks from childhood throughout adolescence and into adulthood intervention strategies targeting PA at young ages will be addressed as well.

THE REGULATION OF ENERGY BALANCE

The continued rise in global obesity rates (NCD Risk Factor Collaboration 2016 and 2017), despite considerable efforts, reflects the limited understanding of the complex interaction of genetic, biochemical, metabolic, psychosocial and cultural factors contributing to the regulation of energy balance. While there remains considerable debate over the contribution of genes, the environment and personal choices to excess body weight, weight gain is ultimately the result of an imbalance between energy expenditure and energy intake (Speakman 2004). Based on the laws of thermodynamics energy expenditure and energy intake need to match over time in order to maintain body weight. A simple opposition of energy expenditure and energy intake, however, ignores the complex interaction between these correlates of energy balance. As shown in Figure 1 there are various feedback mechanisms, where a change in one entity affects other components contributing to energy balance. Participation in PA, for example, affects energy storage, appetite and potentially dietary intake. Increased participation in resistance exercise along with appropriate dietary intake has been shown to increase lean body mass rather than fat mass (Schwingshackl et al. 2013, Collins et al. 2018). An energy surplus at low levels of PA and exercise, on the other hand, most likely results in an increase in body fat. The effects of an energy deficit on body composition also differ by PA and exercise levels. Caloric restriction in non-exercisers has been associated with a greater loss of lean body mass. Exercise associated with caloric restriction, on the other hand, has been shown to induce fat loss, while maintaining lean body mass (Koehler, De Souza, and Williams 2017, Thomas et al. 2012, Weinheimer, Sands, and Campell 2010). Participation in different exercises also appears to affect appetite sensation and food hedonics (Drenowatz, Evensen, et al. 2017), which could affect caloric intake and energy balance. Similarly, alterations in body weight are associated with changes in resting metabolic rate and energy expenditure of various movements (Hand and Blair 2014) as well as subsequent dietary intake (Klok, Jakobsdottir, and Drent 2007).

Further, it should be considered that a continuous energy expenditure needs to be matched by an episodic energy intake, which results in an almost constant imbalance between these two entities; an energy surplus at the end of a meal and an energy deficit during periods without food consumption, including sleep. The considerable daily variability in energy expenditure (roughly 10%) and energy intake (roughly 25%) may also contribute to the limited ability of the regulation of energy balance over short periods of time (Schoeller and Thomas 2015). Accordingly, even weight stable participants do not match their daily energy expenditure with daily energy intake (Hall et al. 2012, Schoeller and Thomas 2015, Westerterp 2010). Along this line, available research indicates an excess energy intake during the weekend and holidays, resulting in weight gain during these periods (Orsama et al. 2014, Racette et al. 2008, Yanovski et al. 2000), which may be compensated for during weekdays and the remainder of the year (following the holiday season), when participants maintain a stable body weight over prolonged periods of time. These weight fluctuations, however, suggest that social constraints potentially override physiological processes and undermine the potential of behavioral chnages in weight management. Of additional concern is that small discrepancies in energy intake and energy expenditure can result in significant weight gain over time (Hill 2006, Speakman et al. 2011). A commonly observed annual weight gain between 0.5 and 1.0 kg, for example, can be attributed to a sustained energy plus of only 50-100 kcal/day (Hill 2006).

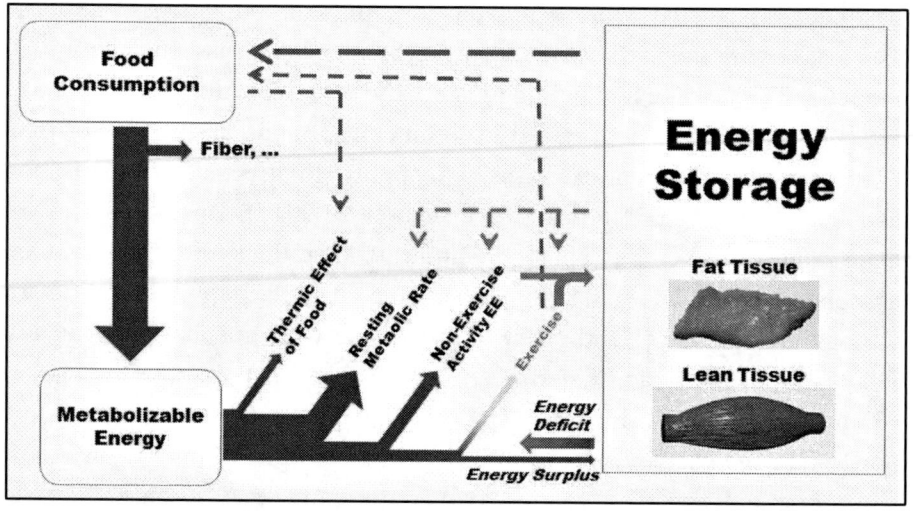

Figure 1. Interaction of dietary intake, energy expenditure and body composition.

Given these limitations along with data from pharmacological weight loss trials the physiological regulation of body weight may be questioned (Müller, Bosy-Westphal, and Heymsfield 2010). Rather, the rate of energy intake and energy expenditure, which is referred to as energy flux, has been suggested to play an important role in weight management (Hill, Wyatt, and Peters 2012, Drenowatz, Hill, et al. 2017, Hand and Blair 2014). While energy balance can theoretically be achieved at various levels of energy flux (i.e., low energy intake matched by low energy expenditure or high energy intake matched by high energy expenditure), available research indicates a better regulation of energy intake and energy expenditure at higher energy flux (Blundell et al. 2015, Shook et al. 2015, Mayer, Roy, and Mitra 1956). This may be attributed to the fact that human physiology evolved under circumstances of high levels of PA and energy expenditure when energy intake was driven by high energy requirements (Hill, Wyatt, and Peters 2012). Accordingly, PA appears to play a critical role in weight management and general health.

The Role of Physical Activity and Exercise in the Regulation of Energy Balance

In general, a high energy flux is associated with greater PA. Increased body weight, however, provides a viable option to increase energy flux, at lower activity levels (Hand and Blair 2014). In fact, a study in Indian mill workers indicated more than half a century ago that men in sedentary occupations consumed a similar amount of calories as those engaging in heavy work (i.e., blacksmiths, cutters, carriers), which would suggest a similar energy flux (Mayer, Roy, and Mitra 1956). Body weight, however, was significantly higher in those with sedentary occupations. More recent studies also showed similar total daily energy expenditure in adults following a traditional foraging or farming lifestyle, characterized by high PA levels, and those living a typical western lifestyle, characterized by predominantly sedentary habits (Pontzer et al. 2012, Esparza et al. 2000). Further, Dugas et al. (2011) reported no difference in total daily energy expenditure between populations living in low, middle, or highly developed countries. There are, however, considerable differences in body weight and body composition between these populations with a higher body weight and body fat in western societies that are characterized by a sedentary lifestyle.

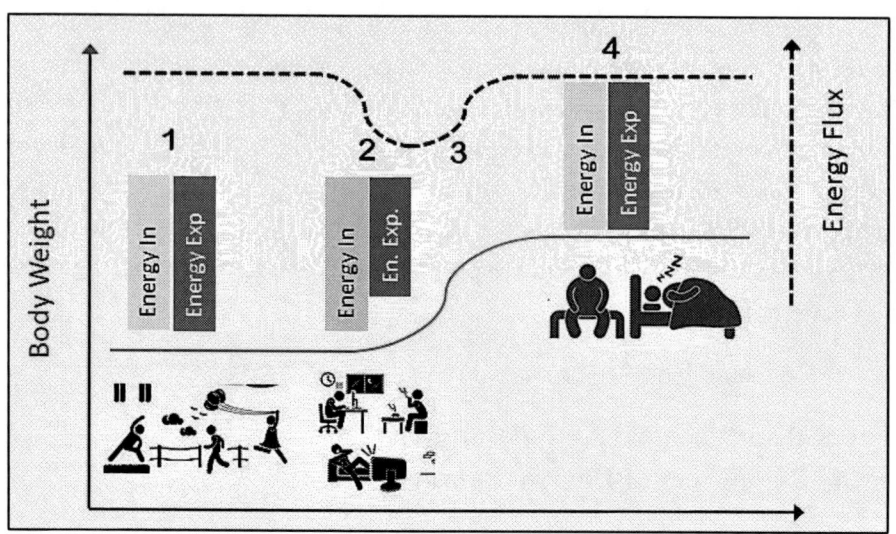

Figure 2. Interaction of physical activity and body weight in the regulation of energy flux.
1. stable energy flux with healthy body weight and high physical activity; 2 reduction of physical activity – due to decline in energy expenditure imbalance with energy intake; 3. weight gain due to positive energy balance with associated increase in energy expenditure; 4 stable energy flux due with high body weight and low physical activity.

As has been observed across different populations there also appears to be limited change in daily energy expenditure at the individual level despite significant alterations in body weight (Drenowatz, Hill, et al. 2017). While weight change is certainly associated with short-term alterations in energy expenditure and energy intake, these alterations may be small in nature and, therefore, difficult to detect. More obvious changes, however, were observed in behavioral choices. Participants who lost weight displayed a significant increase in time spent in moderate-to-vigorous PA (MVPA), while participants who gained weight reduced their time spent in MVPA (Drenowatz, Hill, et al. 2017). Data from monozygotic twins also did not show significant differences in energy expenditure and energy intake despite considerable differences in body weight and PA level (Pietiläinen et al. 2010, Doornweerd et al. 2016).

It can, therefore, be speculated that energy flux, rather than energy balance is a regulated entity. Human beings, however, can use different strategies to maintain their energy flux – high levels of PA at low body weight or high body weight at low PA levels (Figure 2). The detrimental effects of excess body weight on health and well-being (Reilly et al. 2003, Lobstein et al. 2004), however, suggest that PA should be emphasized as important component in the long-term regulation of body weight and energy balance.

The importance of PA for the regulation of energy balance and body weight may be attributed to the fact that participation in PA was necessary for survival and, accordingly, has been considered a biologically normal condition in pre-industrial areas (Booth and Lees 2006, Hawley and Holloszy 2009). A limited and insecure food supply during these times may further have contributed to a predisposition for overeating and an efficient energy storage in the form of body fat when excess food was available in order to prepare for times when food was sparse (Chakravarthy and Booth 2004). The easy access to food in the modern environment without the necessity of high PA, however, contributes to a mismatch between physiology and environment that facilitates weight gain. Human beings, unfortunately display limited biological regulation against overconsumption while they have developed biological adaptations for hunger (Peters et al. 2002, Heitmann et al. 2012). Further, there appear to be biological defense mechanisms to avoid energy deficits (Greenway 2015). Accordingly, weight gain can be viewed as normal and predictable adaptation in response to a sedentary lifestyle as this increases energy expenditure and energy flux at low PA levels. High levels of PA, on the other hand, appear to be necessary in order to maintain a healthy body weight, which has been shown in participants who were able to maintain their body weight after weight loss for a prolonged period of time (Catenacci and Wyatt 2007, Catenacci et al. 2008). Nevertheless, energy flux may differ across individuals and these inter-individual variability may also help to explain the considerable differences in body weight between human beings in similar environments.

PROMOTION OF PHYSICAL ACTIVITY

Despite the well-documented benefits of PA for a variety of health outcomes, including weight management, a large amount of people do not meet current PA recommendations (Guthold et al. 2018). Low PA levels are already reported in children and adolescents and approximately 80% of 13-15-year-olds are considered insufficiently active (Hallal et al. 2012, Cooper et al. 2015, Guthold et al. 2020). Various health-policy statements, therefore, emphasize the importance of sufficient PA and argue for the continued promotion of an active lifestyle (Kahlmeier et al. 2015, US Department of Health and Services 2018, World Health Organization 2010). As lack of time is a commonly cited reason for low PA, strategies targeting the implementation of PA in daily activities may provide better success rates. Active travel, for example, has been considered a viable option to increase PA levels. Available data, however, suggests that the contribution of active travel to total daily energy expenditure is negligible and it has been argued that the general population is unlikely to achieve the necessary volume of locomotor activities that significantly affect daily energy expenditure (Ohkawara et al. 2011, Csizmadi et al. 2011). Rather, higher intensities appear to be necessary to affect body weight and body composition (Boutcher 2011, Trapp et al. 2008, Wareham, van Sluijs, and Ekelund 2005). Accordingly, a more structured approach, including exercise seems necessary.

Traditional exercise interventions, which rely predominantly on aerobic exercise, however, have commonly been of limited success (Dhurandhar et al. 2015). In addition to problems with compliance to the exercise program, this has been attributed to compensatory reductions in habitual PA, which minimizes exercise-induced alterations in energy expenditure (Drenowatz 2015, Westerterp 2001). Resistance exercise, on the other hand, has been associated with an increase in habitual PA, which was, at least partly, attributed to an increased functional capacity (Drenowatz, Grieve, and DeMello 2015, Strasser and Schobersberger 2011). Particularly at young ages, physical fitness and motor competence could be important aspects in the promotion of an active lifestyle as these entities facilitate engagement in various forms of PA (Drenowatz 2017). In fact it has been argued that the lack of sustainable results of exercise interventions may be attributed to limited attention towards physical fitness and motor competence (Cattuzzo et al. 2016, Rodrigues, Stodden, and Lopes 2016). In general, intervention strategies targeting an active lifestyle should facilitate participation in various activities, including habitual PA, as this may allow participants to maintain higher PA levels after the cessation of the intervention. As physical fitness is defined as the ability to carry out daily tasks without undue fatigue and sufficient energy reserves to engage in leisure-time PA (Gallahue, Ozmun and Godway 2012), physical fitness should be considered an important component in the promotion of an active lifestyle.

Promotion of Physicl Activity in Children and Adolescents

The high prevalence of insufficiently active children and adolescents is of particular concern (Tremblay et al. 2016), as PA and sports participation tracks from childhood into adolescence and adulthood (Telama et al. 2014, Richards et al. 2007). Further, the decline in PA is particularly pronounced during childhood and adolescence (Farooq et al. 2018), which is also the age range with the most pronounced increase in the prevalence of overweight and obesity (Hoffmann, Rolf, and Perikles 2012). In addition, it has been argued that attitudes and various behavioral patterns are established during adolescence and that children are more responsive to PA interventions, which could allow for more sustainable effects (Nelson, Neumark-Stzainer, and Sirard 2006). On average, children also display higher PA levels than adults if they are given the opportunity and, therefore, it may be sufficient to focus on maintaining PA at young ages rather than trying to increase activity levels later in life (Drenowatz 2013). Various policy documents, therefore, emphasized the need for effective intervention strategies in children and adolescents (van Sluijs, McMinn, and Griffin 2007).

Common approaches for the promotion of PA in youth include education on the benefits of PA, environmental facilitation, specific structured and supervised activities as well as a combination of these strategies (Drenowatz 2013). Education-based intervention strategies rely on the distribution of information on an active and healthy lifestyle via schools, public media, and health-care providers (e.g., (Patrick et al. 2006, Black et al. 2010, Gentile et al. 2009). Environmental facilitation may include the promotion of active transport, the availability of equipment and safe places for PA during and after school as well as free access to activity facilities (e.g., (Boarnet et al. 2005, Ridgers et al. 2007, de Barros et al. 2009, Verstraete et al. 2007). Specific activity programs commonly relied on active breaks during class-time in schools (e.g., (Pangrazi et al. 2003, Dreyhaupt et al. 2012, Salmon et al. 2011, Graf and Dordel 2011), increased physical education or mandatory PA in after-school programs (e.g., (Sollerhed and Ejlertsson 2008, Gutin et al. 2008, Weintraub et al. 2008). These approaches, however, were of limited success and the evidence on long-term sustainability remains scarce (Drenowatz et al. 2013, Metcalf, Henley, and Wilkin 2012).

Regarding intervention settings, schools have been commonly used for the promotion of PA in children and adolescents as this allows to reach a large number of the target population independent of their socio-economic background (Love, Adams, and van Sluijs 2019). It has further been argued that adolescents are more active during the school day compared to weekends or evening hours (Fairclough, Ridgers, and Welk 2012). Nevertheless, other settings, including family and the community, should be included in order to achieve sustainable intervention effects. Community-based interventions commonly rely on structural changes that facilitate PA (e.g., opportunities for active transport, safe play spaces) but they could also include peer support (Drenowatz et al. 2013, van Sluijs, McMinn, and Griffin 2007). In addition, duration of the intervention period needs to be considered independent of the research setting and strategy. Available research suggests that daily engagement with the intervention over at least one year or repeated interventions over shorter periods are required to increase the likelihood of sustainable effects (Kriemler et al. 2011, van Sluijs and McMinn 2010). These aspects also support the use of schools in the promotion of an active lifestyle as this would provide opportunities for repeated interventions across several years. There are, however, also several aspects that mediate intervention effects, particularly when a group-based approach is taken. Physical fitness and motor competence appear to be particularly important mediators for increased PA, as higher motor competence and physical fitness increases the motivation towards PA and facilitates participation in PA (Robinson et al. 2015). These entities also track moderately from childhood into adolescence (Lima et al. 2017) and are considered sustainable outcomes that could induce permanent change in a person's behavioral capability and preferences for specific lifestyle choices, including PA, during adulthood (Barnett et al. 2009, Lai et al. 2014).

The Role of Physical Fitness and Motor Competence in the Promotion of Physical Activity and Healthy Body Weight

Physical fitness and motor competence are critical determinants in the general development of children and adolescents as they affect physical, psychological and mental health along with overall well-being (Robinson et al. 2015, Cantell, Crawford, and Tish Doyle-Baker 2008, Stodden et al. 2014, Bremer and Cairney 2016). Motor competence is defined as a person's ability to execute various motor tasks required to manage everyday tasks (Vedul-Kjelsås et al. 2012). Along with physical fitness it provides the foundation for specialized movement skills that facilitate participation in sports and active leisure activities (Gallahue, Ozmun, and Goodway 2012). Accordingly, it has been argued that strategies targeting PA and weight management should initially address deficiencies in physical fitness and motor competence as this would facilitate a successful participation in various forms of PA (Cliff et al. 2012, Okely, Booth, and Chey 2004). Higher physial fitness and motor competence have been associated with increased enjoyment of PA and motivation towards an active lifestyle (Barnett et al. 2009, Lopes et al. 2012), which potentially contributes to a lower age-related decline in PA during childhood and adolescence. Further, motor competence and physical fitness during childhood were associated with higher MVPA in adults (Holfelder and Schott 2014).

Even though rudimentary movement patterns develop naturally, there needs to be a conscious effort to facilitate motor development (Hardy et al. 2012). The promotion of motor competence requires practice that consists of free play and structured exercise with appropriate instruction, encouragement and feedback (Gallahue, Ozmun, and Goodway 2012, Robinson and Goodway 2009, Logan et al. 2012). Similarly, improvement in physical fitness requires deliberate practice over a prolonged period of time (Gibson, Wagner and Hayward 2019). Accordingly, there is a reciprocal, synergistic relationship between motor competence, physical fitness and PA, which is also associated with body weight (Hume et al. 2008, Kambas et al. 2012, Stodden et al. 2008). The directionality and strength of the association between motor competence and PA, however, varies by age (Stodden et al. 2008). At younger ages a variety of movement experiences are a prerequisite for the development of motor competence and higher levels of PA will contribute to increased physical fitness. During late childhood and adolescence, perceived and actual motor competence along with physical fitness, however, become major determinants for participation in PA, particularly once children start to compare their abilities to their peers. Higher PA during adolescence further enhances motor competence and physical fitness, which increases the likelihood for sustained participation in exercise and PA during adolescence and into adulthood (Stodden et al. 2008, Barnett et al. 2016). Low motor competence, on the other hand, results in less pleasant movement experiences, which reduces the motivation to engage in challenging activities that would contribute to the improvement of motor competence and physical fitness (Williams et al. 2008, Rose, Larkin, and Berger 1998).

The association between motor competence, physical fitness and PA also affects body weight over time. Longitudinal data has shown positive trajectories of healthy body weight with increased motor performance, while there was an increased risk for overweight and obesity with low motor competence (Stodden, Langendorfer, and Roberton 2009, D'Hondt et al. 2013, Barnett et al. 2009, Lopes et al. 2011). In addition, there is evidence that motor competence and physical fitness affects body composition independent of PA (Lopes et al. 2012). Further, body weight affects motor development as overweight/obesity has been associated with slower motor development and impaired development of physical fitness while weight loss was associated with an augmented motor development and more pronounced improvements in physical fitness (Greier and Drenowatz 2018, Albrecht et al. 2016). In order to avoid a vicious cycle of low PA, low motor performance (including physical fitness and motor competence) and increased body weight, intervention efforts should start at young ages when discrepancies in these components are less pronounced and participants pay less attention towards their peers (Pietiläinen et al. 2008). Children may also experience improvements more quickly as the central nervous system, which plays a critical role in motor development, is more plastic at younger ages (Malina et al. 2004).

In addition, muscle strengthening activities may provide a viable strategy for enhancing PA, particularly in overweight and obese youth as these may allow them to excel in such exercises due to their greater absolute strength as a result of their higher body weight (Ten Hoor et al. 2016). Further, low muscular strength in youth has been associated with an increased risk for functional limitations that may contribute to low PA (Faigenbaum and McFarland 2016, Steene-Johannessen et al. 2009). Nevertheless, there remain reservations towards the implementation of resistance training in pediatric populations (ten Hoor et al. 2015) even though the benefits have been well documented (Faigenbaum and Myer 2010, Mühlbauer et al. 2013). An important part for the implementation of strength training at younger ages, however, is to emphasize movement technique along with a developmentally appropriate progression in intensity (Drenowatz and Greier 2018). A stronger emphasis on motor recruitment and movement technique at young ages also promotes motor development in general. In addition to the positive effects on physical fitness, participation in various resistance exercises broadens movement experience, which has beneficial effects on motor competence and, thus, contributes to the promotion of an active and healthy lifestyle.

CONCLUSION

Low PA along with low physical fitness, poor motor competence and excess body weight are considered major threats to future public health (World Health Organization 2010, Jakicic 2009). Of particular concern is the fact that PA levels remain low and overweight and obesity rates continue to increase despite considerable efforts (Guthold et al. 2018, NCD-Risk Factor Collaboration 2017). These developments may also reflect the limited understanding of key correlates of PA and body weight. The research presented in chapter addressed some key issues regarding the regulation of body weight and the promotion of PA, particularly in children and adolescents with a special emphasis on the role of physical fitness and motor competence.

Even though weight gain is ultimately the result of an imbalance between energy expenditure and energy intake, the large variability in energy expenditure and energy intake may question a biological regulation of energy balance (Schoeller and Thomas 2015, Drenowatz, Hill, et al. 2017). Rather, energy flux, may need to be considered as a regulated entity. This concept also reflects the complex interaction of body weight, energy expenditure and energy intake including a gene-environment interaction (Speakman et al. 2011), rather than the reliance on a simple opposition of energy expenditure and energy intake with body weight as outcome. A regulated energy flux further allows for different strategies to achieve a certain level of energy expenditure which is matched by energy intake and could help to explain the variability in body weight across human beings living in similar environments. People may rely on a certain amount of PA to achieve their predetermined energy expenditure or they may increase their body weight in order to increase energy expenditure in the absence of sufficient PA. Accordingly, PA appears to be a critical component in the regulation of a healthy body weight in addition to general health and well-being.

PA requirements in highly developed societies, however, are limited and people need to make conscious efforts to ensure sufficient PA. Accordingly, various intervention strategies including education, environmental facilitation and exercise programs have been implemented to increase PA (Drenowatz et al. 2013). The success of these strategies, particularly regarding sustainability, however, has been limited. Given the direct association of PA with physical fitness and motor competence (Logan et al. 2015, Robinson et al. 2015), these aspects should be consdiered more strongly in the development of intervention strategies. Both, physical fitness and motor competence facilitate participation in various forms of PA and, therefore, have been suggested as an important components in the promotion of an active lifestyle (Cliff et al. 2012, Okely, Booth, and Chey 2004, Cattuzzo et al. 2016, Rodrigues, Stodden, and Lopes 2016). Emphasizing physical fitness and motor development at young ages by providing a variety of movement experiences, including free play and structured exercise, therefore, appears to be a viable option in the promotion of an active lifestyle. Targeting children and adolescents may further increase the chances for sustainable intervention effects as various behavioral patterns are established during childhood and adolescence (Nelson, Neumark-Stzainer, and Sirard 2006). Even at older ages a focus on physical fitness and motor competence may provide a viable option for the promotion of PA and healthy body weight. More research, however, is necessary to enhance the understanding of the regulation of energy balance and the role of physical fitness and motor competence in the promotion of PA in order to develop intervention strategies targeting an active and healthy lifestyle.

REFERENCES

Albrecht, C, A Hanssen-Doose, D Oriwol, K Bös, and A Worth. 2016. "Beeinflusst ein Veränderung des BMI die Entwicklung der motorischen Leistungsfähigkeit im Kindes- und Jugendalter? Ergebnisse der Motorik-Modul Studie (MoMo)." *Bewegungstherapie und Gesundheitssport 32:*168-172. [Does a change in BMI affect the development of motor performance in children and adolescents? Results of the Motor Skills Module Study (MoMo). *Exercise therapy and health sports*]

Archer, E., R. P. Shook, D. M. Thomas, T. S. Church, P. T. Katzmarzyk, J. R. Hébert, K. L. McIver, G. A. Hand, C. J. Lavie, and S. N. Blair. 2013. "45-Year trends in women's use of time and household management energy expenditure." *PLoS One 8 (2):*e56620.

Barnett, L. M., S. K. Lai, S. L. Veldman, L. L. Hardy, D. P. Cliff, P. J. Morgan, A. Zask, D. R. Lubans, S. P. Shultz, N. D. Ridgers, E. Rush, H. L. Brown, and A. D. Okely. 2016. "Correlates of Gross Motor Competence in Children and Adolescents: A Systematic Review and Meta-Analysis." *Sports Med 46 (11):*1663-1688.

Barnett, L. M., E. van Beurden, P. J. Morgan, L. O. Brooks, and J. R. Beard. 2009. "Childhood motor skill proficiency as a predictor of adolescent physical activity." *J Adolesc Health 44 (3):*252-259.

Biddle, S. J. H., E. García Bengoechea, Z. Pedisic, J. Bennie, I. Vergeer, and G. Wiesner. 2017. "Screen Time, Other Sedentary Behaviours, and Obesity Risk in Adults: A Review of Reviews." *Curr Obes Rep 6 (2):*134-147.

Black, M. M., E. R. Hager, K. Le, J. Anliker, S. S. Arteaga, C. Diclemente, J. Gittelsohn, L. Magder, M. Papas, S. Snitker, M. S. Treuth, and Y. Wang. 2010. "Challenge! Health promotion/obesity prevention mentorship model among urban, black adolescents." *Pediatrics 126 (2):*280-288.

Blundell, J. E., C. Gibbons, P. Caudwell, G. Finlayson, and M. Hopkins. 2015. "Appetite control and energy balance: impact of exercise." *Obes Rev 16 Suppl 1:*67-76.

Boarnet, M. G., C. L. Anderson, K. Day, T. McMillan, and M. Alfonzo. 2005. "Evaluation of the California Safe Routes to School legislation: urban form changes and children's active transportation to school." *Am J Prev Med 28 (2 Suppl 2):*134-140.

Booth, F. W., and S. J. Lees. 2006. "Physically active subjects should be the control group." *Med Sci Sports Exerc 38 (3):*405-406.

Boutcher, S. H. 2011. "High-intensity intermittent exercise and fat loss." *J Obes 2011:*868305.

Bremer, E, and J Cairney. 2016. "Fundamental movement skills and health-related outcomes: A narrative review of longitudinal and intervention studies targeting typically developing children." *Am J Lifestyle Med 12(2):* 148-159.

Bryant, E. S., M. J. Duncan, and S. L. Birch. 2014. "Fundamental movement skills and weight status in British primary school children." *Eur J Sport Sci 14 (7):*730-736.

Brønnum-Hansen, H., K. Juel, M. Davidsen, and J. Sørensen. 2007. "Impact of selected risk factors on expected lifetime without long-standing, limiting illness in Denmark." *Prev Med 45 (1):*49-53.

Cantell, M., S. G. Crawford, and P. K. Tish Doyle-Baker. 2008. "Physical fitness and health indices in children, adolescents and adults with high or low motor competence." *Hum Mov Sci 27 (2):*344-362.

Catenacci, V. A., L. G. Ogden, J. Stuht, S. Phelan, R. R. Wing, J. O. Hill, and H. R. Wyatt. 2008. "Physical activity patterns in the National Weight Control Registry." *Obesity (Silver Spring) 16 (1):*153-161.

Catenacci, V. A., and H. R. Wyatt. 2007. "The role of physical activity in producing and maintaining weight loss." *Nat Clin Pract Endocrinol Metab 3 (7):*518-529.

Cattuzzo, M. T., R. Dos Santos Henrique, A. H. Ré, I. S. de Oliveira, B. M. Melo, M. de Sousa Moura, R. C. de Araújo, and D. Stodden. 2016. "Motor competence and health related physical fitness in youth: A systematic review." *J Sci Med Sport 19 (2):*123-129.

Chakravarthy, MV, and FW Booth. 2004. "Eating, exercise and "thrifty" genotypes: connecting the dots toward an evolutionary understanding of modern chronic diseases." *J Appl Physiol 96:*3-10.

Church, T. S., D. M. Thomas, C. Tudor-Locke, P. T. Katzmarzyk, C. P. Earnest, R. Q. Rodarte, C. K. Martin, S. N. Blair, and C. Bouchard. 2011. "Trends over 5 decades in U.S. occupation-related physical activity and their associations with obesity." *PLoS One 6 (5):*e19657.

Cliff, D. P., A. D. Okely, P. J. Morgan, R. A. Jones, J. R. Steele, and L. A. Baur. 2012. "Proficiency deficiency: mastery of fundamental movement skills and skill components in overweight and obese children." *Obesity (Silver Spring) 20 (5):*1024-1033.

Collins, H, S Fawkner, JN Booth, and A Duncan. 2018. "The effect of resistance training interventions on weight status in youth: a meta-analysis." *Sports Medicine - Open 4:*41.

Cooper, A. R., A. Goodman, A. S. Page, L. B. Sherar, D. W. Esliger, E. M. van Sluijs, L. B. Andersen, S. Anderssen, G. Cardon, R. Davey, K. Froberg, P. Hallal, K. F. Janz, K. Kordas, S. Kreimler, R. R. Pate, J. J. Puder, J. J. Reilly, J. Salmon, L. B. Sardinha, A. Timperio, and U. Ekelund. 2015. "Objectively measured physical activity and sedentary time in youth: the International children's accelerometry database (ICAD)." *Int J Behav Nutr Phys Act 12:*113.

Csizmadi, I., G. Lo Siou, C. M. Friedenreich, N. Owen, and P. J. Robson. 2011. "Hours spent and energy expended in physical activity domains: results from the Tomorrow Project cohort in Alberta, Canada." *Int J Behav Nutr Phys Act 8:*110.

D'Hondt, E., B. Deforche, I. Gentier, I. De Bourdeaudhuij, R. Vaeyens, R. Philippaerts, and M. Lenoir. 2013. "A longitudinal analysis of gross motor coordination in overweight and obese children versus normal-weight peers." *Int J Obes (Lond) 37 (1):*61-67.

de Barros, M. V., M. V. Nahas, P. C. Hallal, J. C. de Farias Júnior, A. A. Florindo, and S. S. Honda de Barros. 2009. "Effectiveness of a school-based intervention on physical activity for high school students in Brazil: the Saude na Boa project." *J Phys Act Health 6 (2):*163-169.

Dhurandhar, E. J., K. A. Kaiser, J. A. Dawson, A. S. Alcorn, K. D. Keating, and D. B. Allison. 2015. "Predicting adult weight change in the real world: a systematic review and meta-analysis accounting for compensatory changes in energy intake or expenditure." *Int J Obes (Lond) 39 (8):*1181-1187.

Dollman, J., K. Norton, and L. Norton. 2005. "Evidence for secular trends in children's physical activity behaviour." *Br J Sports Med 39 (12):*892-897.

Doornweerd, S., R. G. IJzerman, L. van der Eijk, J. E. Neter, J. van Dongen, H. P. van der Ploeg, and E. J. de Geus. 2016. "Physical activity and dietary intake in BMI discordant identical twins." *Obesity (Silver Spring) 24 (6):*1349-1355.

Drenowatz, C. 2013. "Strategies for physical activity intervention in youth." *J Behav Health 2 (2):*189-196.

Drenowatz, C. 2017. "A focus on motor competence as alternative strategy for weight management." *J Obes Chron Dis 1 (2):*31-38.

Drenowatz, C, and K Greier. 2018. "Implementation of strength training in youth: benefits and considerations." In *Advances in health and disease,* edited by LT Duncan, 149-176. New York, NY: Nova Science Publishers, Inc.

Drenowatz, C, O Wartha, N Fischbach, and JM Steinacker. 2013. "Intervention strategies for the promotion of physical activity in youth." *Dtsch Z Sportmed 64:*170-175.

Drenowatz, C. 2015. "Reciprocal Compensation to Changes in Dietary Intake and Energy Expenditure within the Concept of Energy Balance." *Adv Nutr 6 (5):*592-599.

Drenowatz, C., L. H. Evensen, L. Ernstsen, J. E. Blundell, G. A. Hand, R. P. Shook, J. R. Hébert, S. Burgess, and S. N. Blair. 2017. "Cross-sectional and longitudinal associations between different exercise types and food cravings in free-living healthy young adults." *Appetite 118:*82-89.

Drenowatz, C., G. L. Grieve, and M. M. DeMello. 2015. "Change in energy expenditure and physical activity in response to aerobic and resistance exercise programs." *Springerplus 4:*798.

Drenowatz, C., J. O. Hill, J. C. Peters, A. Soriano-Maldonado, and S. N. Blair. 2017. "The association of change in physical activity and body weight in the regulation of total energy expenditure." *Eur J Clin Nutr 71 (3):*377-382.

Dreyhaupt, J., B. Koch, T. Wirt, A. Schreiber, S. Brandstetter, D. Kesztyues, O. Wartha, S. Kobel, S. Kettner, D. Prokopchuk, V. Hundsdoerfer, M. Klepsch, M. Wiedom, S. Sufeida, N. Fischbach, R. Muche, T. Seufert, and J. M. Steinacker. 2012. "Evaluation of a health promotion program in children: Study protocol and design of the cluster-randomized Baden-Wuerttemberg primary school study." *BMC Public Health 12 (1):*157.

Dugas, L. R., R. Harders, S. Merrill, K. Ebersole, D. A. Shoham, E. C. Rush, F. K. Assah, T. Forrester, R. A. Durazo-Arvizu, and A. Luke. 2011.

"Energy expenditure in adults living in developing compared with industrialized countries: a meta-analysis of doubly labeled water studies." *Am J Clin Nutr 93 (2):*427-441.

Esparza, J., C. Fox, I. T. Harper, P. H. Bennett, L. O. Schulz, M. E. Valencia, and E. Ravussin. 2000. "Daily energy expenditure in Mexican and USA Pima Indians: low physical activity as a possible cause of obesity." *Int J Obes Relat Metab Disord 24 (1):*55-9.

Faigenbaum, A. D., and G. D. Myer. 2010. "Pediatric resistance training: benefits, concerns, and program design considerations." *Curr Sports Med Rep 9 (3):*161-168.

Faigenbaum, AD, and JE McFarland. 2016. "Resistance training for kids: right from the start." *ACSM's Health and Fitness Journal 20 (5):*16-22.

Fairclough, S. J., N. D. Ridgers, and G. Welk. 2012. "Correlates of children's moderate and vigorous physical activity during weekdays and weekends." *J Phys Act Health 9 (1):*129-137.

Farooq, M. A., K. N. Parkinson, A. J. Adamson, M. S. Pearce, J. K. Reilly, A. R. Hughes, X. Janssen, L. Basterfield, and J. J. Reilly. 2018. "Timing of the decline in physical activity in childhood and adolescence: Gateshead Millennium Cohort Study." *Br J Sports Med 52 (15):*1002-1006.

Finkelstein, E. A., O. A. Khavjou, H. Thompson, J. G. Trogdon, L. Pan, B. Sherry, and W. Dietz. 2012. "Obesity and severe obesity forecasts through 2030." *Am J Prev Med 42 (6):*563-570.

Flegal, K. M., M. D. Carroll, C. L. Ogden, and L. R. Curtin. 2010. "Prevalence and trends in obesity among US adults, 1999-2008." *JAMA 303 (3):*235-241.

Gallahue, D, J Ozmun, and J Goodway. 2012. *Understanding Motor Development. Infants, Children, Adolescents, Adults. 7th Ed*. ed. Boston, MA: McGraw-Hill.

Gentile, D. A., G. Welk, J. C. Eisenmann, R. A. Reimer, D. A. Walsh, D. W. Russell, R. Callahan, M. Walsh, S. Strickland, and K. Fritz. 2009. "Evaluation of a multiple ecological level child obesity prevention program: Switch what you Do, View, and Chew." *BMC Med 7:*49.

Gibson, A. L., D. R. Wagner, and V. H. Hayward. 2019. "*Advanced fitness assessment and exercise prescription, 8th Ed.*" Champaign, IL: Human Kinetics.

Goodway, J. D., L. E. Robinson, and H. Crowe. 2010. "Gender differences in fundamental motor skill development in disadvantaged preschoolers from two geographical regions." *Res Q Exerc Sport 81 (1):*17-24.

Graf, C., and S. Dordel. 2011. "[The CHILT I project (Children's Health Interventional Trial). A multicomponent intervention to prevent physical inactivity and overweight in primary schools]." *Bundesgesundheitsblatt Gesundheitsforschung Gesundheitsschutz 54 (3):*313-321.

Greier, K., and C. Drenowatz. 2018. "Bidirectional association between weight status and motor skills in adolescents: A 4-year longitudinal study." *Wien Klin Wochenschr 130 (9-10):*314-320.

Guthold, R., G. A. Stevens, L. M. Riley, and F. C. Bull. 2018. "Worldwide trends in insufficient physical activity from 2001 to 2016: a pooled analysis of 358 population-based surveys with 1·9 million participants." *Lancet Glob Health 6 (10):*e1077-e1086.

Guthold, R., G. A. Stevens, L. M. Riley, and F. C. Bull. 2020. "Global trends in insufficient physical activity among adolescents: a pooloed analysis of 298 population-based surveys with 1.6 million participants." *Lanced Child Adolesc Health 4:* 23-35.

Gutin, B., Z. Yin, M. Johnson, and P. Barbeau. 2008. "Preliminary findings of the effect of a 3-year after-school physical activity intervention on fitness and body fat: the Medical College of Georgia Fitkid Project." *Int J Pediatr Obes 3 Suppl 1:*3-9.

Hall, K. D. 2018. "Did the Food Environment Cause the Obesity Epidemic?" *Obesity (Silver Spring) 26 (1):*11-13.

Hall, K. D., S. B. Heymsfield, J. W. Kemnitz, S. Klein, D. A. Schoeller, and J. R. Speakman. 2012. "Energy balance and its components: implications for body weight regulation." *Am J Clin Nutr 95 (4):*989-994.

Hallal, P. C., L. B. Andersen, F. C. Bull, R. Guthold, W. Haskell, U. Ekelund, and Lancet Physical Activity Series Working Group. 2012.

"Global physical activity levels: surveillance progress, pitfalls, and prospects." *Lancet 380 (9838):*247-257.

Hand, GA, and SN Blair. 2014. "Energy flux and its role in obesity and metabolic disease." *US Endocrinology 10 (1):*59-64.

Hardy, L. L., L. Barnett, P. Espinel, and A. D. Okely. 2013. "Thirteen-year trends in child and adolescent fundamental movement skills: 1997-2010." *Med Sci Sports Exerc 45 (10):*1965-1970.

Hardy, L. L., T. Reinten-Reynolds, P. Espinel, A. Zask, and A. D. Okely. 2012. "Prevalence and correlates of low fundamental movement skill competency in children." *Pediatrics 130 (2):*e390-398.

Hawley, J. A., and J. O. Holloszy. 2009. "Exercise: it's the real thing!" *Nutr Rev 67 (3):*172-178.

Heitmann, B. L., K. R. Westerterp, R. J. Loos, T. I. Sørensen, K. O'Dea, P. McLean, T. K. Jensen, J. Eisenmann, J. R. Speakman, S. J. Simpson, D. R. Reed, and M. S. Westerterp-Plantenga. 2012. "Obesity: lessons from evolution and the environment." *Obes Rev 13 (10):*910-922.

Hill, J. O. 2006. "Understanding and addressing the epidemic of obesity: an energy balance perspective." *Endocr Rev 27 (7):*750-761.

Hill, J. O., H. R. Wyatt, and J. C. Peters. 2012. "Energy balance and obesity." *Circulation 126 (1):*126-132.

Hill, J. O., H. R. Wyatt, G. W. Reed, and J. C. Peters. 2003. "Obesity and the environment: where do we go from here?" *Science 299 (5608):*853-855.

Hoffmann, SW, U Rolf, and S Perikles. 2012. "Refined analysis of the critical age ranges of childhood overweight: implications for primary prevention." *Obesity 20 (10):*2151-2154.

Holfelder, B, and N Schott. 2014. "Relationship of fundamental movement skills in physical activity in children and adolescents: A systematic review." Psychology of Sport and Exercise 15:382-391.

Hume, C., A. Okely, S. Bagley, A. Telford, M. Booth, D. Crawford, and J. Salmon. 2008. "Does weight status influence associations between children's fundamental movement skills and physical activity?" *Res Q Exerc Sport 79 (2):*158-165.

Jakicic, J. M. 2009. "The effect of physical activity on body weight." *Obesity (Silver Spring) 17 Suppl 3:*S34-38.

Kahlmeier, S., T. M. Wijnhoven, P. Alpiger, C. Schweizer, J. Breda, and B. W. Martin. 2015. "National physical activity recommendations: systematic overview and analysis of the situation in European countries." *BMC Public Health 15:*133.

Kambas, A., M. Michalopoulou, I. G. Fatouros, C. Christoforidis, E. Manthou, D. Giannakidou, F. Venetsanou, E. Haberer, A. Chatzinikolaou, V. Gourgoulis, and R. Zimmer. 2012. "The relationship between motor proficiency and pedometer-determined physical activity in young children." *Pediatr Exerc Sci 24 (1):*34-44.

Klok, M. D., S. Jakobsdottir, and M. L. Drent. 2007. "The role of leptin and ghrelin in the regulation of food intake and body weight in humans: a review." *Obes Rev 8 (1):*21-34.

Koehler, K., M. J. De Souza, N. I. Williams. 2017. "Less-than-expected weight loss in normal-weight women undergoing caloric restriction and exercise is accompanied by preservation of fat-free mass and metabolic adaptations." *Eur J Clin Nutr 71 (3):* 365-371.

Kohl, H. W., C. L. Craig, E. V. Lambert, S. Inoue, J. R. Alkandari, G. Leetongin, S. Kahlmeier, and Lancet Physical Activity Series Working Group. 2012. "The pandemic of physical inactivity: global action for public health." *Lancet 380 (9838):*294-305.

Kriemler, S., U. Meyer, E. Martin, E. M. van Sluijs, L. B. Andersen, and B. W. Martin. 2011. "Effect of school-based interventions on physical activity and fitness in children and adolescents: a review of reviews and systematic update." *Br J Sports Med 45 (11):*923-930.

Lai, SK, SA Costigan, PJ Morgan, DR Lubans, DF Stodden, J Salmon, and LM Barnett. 2014. "Do school-based interventions focusing on physical activity, fitness, or fundamental movement skill competency produce a sustained impact in these outcomes in children and adolescents? A systematic review of follow-up studies." *Sports Med 44 (1):*67-79.

Lima, R. A., A. Bugge, K. A. Pfeiffer, and L. B. Andersen. 2017. "Tracking of Gross Motor Coordination from Childhood into Adolescence." *Res Q Exerc Sport 88 (1):*52-59.

Lobstein, T., L. Baur, R. Uauy, and IASO International Obesity TaskForce. 2004. "Obesity in children and young people: a crisis in public health." *Obes Rev 5 Suppl 1:*4-104.

Lobstein, T., R. Jackson-Leach, M. L. Moodie, K. D. Hall, S. L. Gortmaker, B. A. Swinburn, W. P. James, Y. Wang, and K. McPherson. 2015. "Child and adolescent obesity: part of a bigger picture." *Lancet 385 (9986):*2510-2520.

Logan, S. W., L. E. Robinson, A. E. Wilson, and W. A. Lucas. 2012. "Getting the fundamentals of movement: a meta-analysis of the effectiveness of motor skill interventions in children." *Child Care Health Dev 38 (3):*305-315.

Logan, SW, K Webster, N Getchell, KA Pfeiffer, and LE Robinson. 2015. "Relationship between fundamental motor skill competence and physical activity during childhood and adolescence: a systematic review." *Kines Rev 4:*416-426.

Lopes, V. P., L. P. Rodrigues, J. A. Maia, and R. M. Malina. 2011. "Motor coordination as predictor of physical activity in childhood." *Scand J Med Sci Sports 21 (5):*663-669.

Lopes, VP, JAR Maia, LP Rodrigues, and R Malina. 2012. "Motor coordination, physical activity and fitness as predictors of longitudinal change in adiposity during childhood." *Eur J Sport Sci 12 (4):*384-391.

Love, R., J. Adams, and E. M. F. van Sluijs. 2019. "Are school-based physical activity interventions effective and equitable? A meta-analysis of cluster randomized controlled trials with accelerometer-assessed activity." *Obes Rev 20(6):*859-870.

Lubans, D., and P. Morgan. 2008. "Evaluation of an extra-curricular school sport programme promoting lifestyle and lifetime activity for adolescents." *J Sports Sci 26 (5):*519-529.

Mayer, J., P. Roy, and K. P. Mitra. 1956. "Relation between caloric intake, body weight, and physical work: studies in an industrial male population in West Bengal." *Am J Clin Nutr 4 (2):*169-175.

Melanson, E. L., S. K. Keadle, J. E. Donnelly, B. Braun, and N. A. King. 2013. "Resistance to exercise-induced weight loss: compensatory behavioral adaptations." *Med Sci Sports Exerc 45 (8):*1600-1609.

Metcalf, B., W. Henley, and T. Wilkin. 2012. "Effectiveness of intervention on physical activity of children: systematic review and meta-analysis of controlled trials with objectively measured outcomes (Early Bird 54)." *BMJ 345:*e5888.

Mühlbauer, T, R Roth, A Kibele, DG Behm, and U Granacher. 2013. Krafttraining mit Kindern und Jugendlichen: Praktische Umsetzung und theoretische Grundlagen [*Strength training with children and adoescents: Practical application and theoretical foundations*]. Schorndorf: Hofmann-Verlag.

Müller, M. J., A. Bosy-Westphal, and S. B. Heymsfield. 2010. "Is there evidence for a set point that regulates human body weight?" *F1000 Med Rep 2:*59.

NCD Risk Factor Collaboration. 2016. "Trends in adult body-mass index in 200 countries from 1975 to 2014: a pooled analysis of 1698 population-based measurement studies with 19·2 million participants." *Lancet 387 (10026):*1377-1396.

NCD Risk Factor Collaboration. 2017. "Worldwide trends in body-mass index, underweight, overweight, and obesity from 1975 to 2016: a pooled analysis of 2416 population-based measurement studies in 128·9 million children, adolescents, and adults." *Lancet 390 (10113):*2627-2642.

Nelson, MC, HJ Neumark-Stzainer, and JR Sirard. 2006. "Longitudinal and secular trends in physical activity and sedentary behavior during adolescence." *Pediatrics 118:*e1627.

O'Brien, W, S Belton, and J Issartel. 2016. "Fundamental movement skill proficiency amongst adolescent youth." *Phys Ed Sport Pedagog 21 (6):*557-571.

O'Donovan, G., A. J. Blazevich, C. Boreham, A. R. Cooper, H. Crank, U. Ekelund, K. R. Fox, P. Gately, B. Giles-Corti, J. M. Gill, M. Hamer, I. McDermott, M. Murphy, N. Mutrie, J. J. Reilly, J. M. Saxton, and E. Stamatakis. 2010. "The ABC of Physical Activity for Health: a consensus statement from the British Association of Sport and Exercise Sciences." *J Sports Sci 28 (6):*573-591.

Ohkawara, K., K. Ishikawa-Takata, J. H. Park, I. Tabata, and S. Tanaka. 2011. "How much locomotive activity is needed for an active physical activity level: analysis of total step counts." *BMC Res Notes 4:*512.

Okely, A. D., M. L. Booth, and T. Chey. 2004. "Relationships between body composition and fundamental movement skills among children and adolescents." *Res Q Exerc Sport 75 (3):*238-247.

Orsama, A. L., E. Mattila, M. Ermes, M. van Gils, B. Wansink, and I. Korhonen. 2014. "Weight rhythms: weight increases during weekends and decreases during weekdays." *Obes Facts 7 (1):*36-47.

Pangrazi, R. P., A. Beighle, T. Vehige, and C. Vack. 2003. "Impact of Promoting Lifestyle Activity for Youth (PLAY) on children's physical activity." *J Sch Health 73 (8):*317-321.

Patrick, K., K. J. Calfas, G. J. Norman, M. F. Zabinski, J. F. Sallis, J. Rupp, J. Covin, and J. Cella. 2006. "Randomized controlled trial of a primary care and home-based intervention for physical activity and nutrition behaviors: PACE+ for adolescents." *Arch Pediatr Adolesc Med 160 (2):*128-136.

Peters, J. C., H. R. Wyatt, W. T. Donahoo, and J. O. Hill. 2002. "From instinct to intellect: the challenge of maintaining healthy weight in the modern world." *Obes Rev 3 (2):*69-74.

Pietiläinen, K. H., J. Kaprio, P. Borg, G. Plasqui, H. Yki-Järvinen, U. M. Kujala, R. J. Rose, K. R. Westerterp, and A. Rissanen. 2008. "Physical inactivity and obesity: a vicious circle." *Obesity (Silver Spring) 16 (2):*409-414.

Pietiläinen, K. H., M. Korkeila, L. H. Bogl, K. R. Westerterp, H. Yki-Järvinen, J. Kaprio, and A. Rissanen. 2010. "Inaccuracies in food and physical activity diaries of obese subjects: complementary evidence from doubly labeled water and co-twin assessments." *Int J Obes (Lond) 34 (3):*437-445.

Pontzer, H., D. A. Raichlen, B. M. Wood, A. Z. Mabulla, S. B. Racette, and F. W. Marlowe. 2012. "Hunter-gatherer energetics and human obesity." *PLoS One 7 (7):*e40503.

Racette, S. B., E. P. Weiss, K. B. Schechtman, K. Steger-May, D. T. Villareal, K. A. Obert, and J. O. Holloszy. 2008. "Influence of weekend lifestyle patterns on body weight." *Obesity (Silver Spring) 16 (8):*1826-1830.

Reilly, J. J., E. Methven, Z. C. McDowell, B. Hacking, D. Alexander, L. Stewart, and C. J. Kelnar. 2003. "Health consequences of obesity." *Arch Dis Child 88 (9):*748-752.

Richards, R., S. Williams, R. Poulton, and A. I. Reeder. 2007. "Tracking club sport participation from childhood to early adulthood." *Res Q Exerc Sport 78 (5):*413-419.

Ridgers, N. D., G. Stratton, S. J. Fairclough, and J. W. Twisk. 2007. "Long-term effects of a playground markings and physical structures on children's recess physical activity levels." *Prev Med 44 (5):*393-397.

Robinson, L. E., and J. D. Goodway. 2009. "Instructional climates in preschool children who are at-risk. Part I: object-control skill development." *Res Q Exerc Sport 80 (3):*533-542.

Robinson, L. E., D. F. Stodden, L. M. Barnett, V. P. Lopes, S. W. Logan, L. P. Rodrigues, and E. D'Hondt. 2015. "Motor Competence and its Effect on Positive Developmental Trajectories of Health." *Sports Med 45 (9):*1273-1284.

Rodrigues, L. P., D. F. Stodden, and V. P. Lopes. 2016. "Developmental pathways of change in fitness and motor competence are related to overweight and obesity status at the end of primary school." *J Sci Med Sport 19 (1):*87-92.

Rose, B, D Larkin, and BG Berger. 1998. "The importance of motor coordination for children's motivational orientations in sport." *Adapt Phys Act Q 15:*316-327.

Roth, K., K. Ruf, M. Obinger, S. Mauer, J. Ahnert, W. Schneider, C. Graf, and H. Hebestreit. 2010. "Is there a secular decline in motor skills in preschool children?" *Scand J Med Sci Sports 20 (4):*670-678.

Salmon, J., L. Arundell, C. Hume, H. Brown, K. Hesketh, D. W. Dunstan, R. M. Daly, N. Pearson, E. Cerin, M. Moodie, L. Sheppard, K. Ball, S. Bagley, M. C. Paw, and D. Crawford. 2011. "A cluster-randomized controlled trial to reduce sedentary behavior and promote physical activity and health of 8-9 year olds: the Transform-Us! study." *BMC Public Health 11:*759.

Schoeller, D. A., and D. Thomas. 2015. "Energy balance and body composition." *World Rev Nutr Diet 111:*13-18.

Schwingshackl, L., S. Dias, B. Strasser, and G. Hoffmann. 2013. "Impact of different training modalities on anthropometric and metabolic characteristics in overweight/obese subjects: a systematic review and network meta-analysis." *PLoS One 8 (12):*e82853.

Shaw, K., H. Gennat, P. O'Rourke, and C. Del Mar. 2006. "Exercise for overweight or obesity." *Cochrane Database Syst Rev (4):*CD003817.

Shook, R. P., G. A. Hand, C. Drenowatz, J. R. Hebert, A. E. Paluch, J. E. Blundell, J. O. Hill, P. T. Katzmarzyk, T. S. Church, and S. N. Blair. 2015. "Low levels of physical activity are associated with dysregulation of energy intake and fat mass gain over 1 year." *Am J Clin Nutr. 102(6):*1332-1338.

Singh, A. S., C. Mulder, J. W. Twisk, W. van Mechelen, and M. J. Chinapaw. 2008. "Tracking of childhood overweight into adulthood: a systematic review of the literature." *Obes Rev 9 (5):*474-488.

Sinha, R., G. Fisch, B. Teague, W. V. Tamborlane, B. Banyas, K. Allen, M. Savoye, V. Rieger, S. Taksali, G. Barbetta, R. S. Sherwin, and S. Caprio. 2002. "Prevalence of impaired glucose tolerance among children and adolescents with marked obesity." *N Engl J Med 346 (11):*802-810.

Sollerhed, A. C., and G. Ejlertsson. 2008. "Physical benefits of expanded physical education in primary school: findings from a 3-year intervention study in Sweden." *Scand J Med Sci Sports 18 (1):*102-107.

Speakman, J. R. 2004. "Obesity: the integrated roles of environment and genetics." *J Nutr 134 (8 Suppl):*2090S-2105S.

Speakman, J. R., D. A. Levitsky, D. B. Allison, M. S. Bray, J. M. de Castro, D. J. Clegg, J. C. Clapham, A. G. Dulloo, L. Gruer, S. Haw, J. Hebebrand, M. M. Hetherington, S. Higgs, S. A. Jebb, R. J. Loos, S. Luckman, A. Luke, V. Mohammed-Ali, S. O'Rahilly, M. Pereira, L. Perusse, T. N. Robinson, B. Rolls, M. E. Symonds, and M. S. Westerterp-Plantenga. 2011. "Set points, settling points and some alternative models: theoretical options to understand how genes and environments combine to regulate body adiposity." *Dis Model Mech 4 (6):*733-745.

Steene-Johannessen, J., S. A. Anderssen, E. Kolle, and L. B. Andersen. 2009. "Low muscle fitness is associated with metabolic risk in youth." Med Sci Sports *Exerc 41 (7)*:1361-1367.

Stodden, D. F., Z. Gao, J. D. Goodway, and S. J. Langendorfer. 2014. "Dynamic relationships between motor skill competence and health-related fitness in youth." Pediatr Exerc *Sci 26 (3):231-41*.

Stodden, D., S. Langendorfer, and M. A. Roberton. 2009. "The association between motor skill competence and physical fitness in young adults." Res Q Exerc S*port 80 (2):223-229*.

Stodden, DF, JD Goodway, SJ Langendorfer, MA Roberton, ME Rudisill, C Garcia, and LE Garcia. 2008. "A developmental perspective on the role of motor skill competence in physical activity: an emergent relationshihp." Quest 60:290-*306*.

Strasser, B., and W. Schobersberger. 2011. "Evidence for resistance training as a treatment therapy in obesity." *J Obes 2011:*482564.

Telama, R., X. Yang, E. Leskinen, A. Kankaanpää, M. Hirvensalo, T. Tammelin, J. S. Viikari, and O. T. Raitakari. 2014. "Tracking of physical activity from early childhood through youth into adulthood." *Med Sci Sports Exerc 46 (5):*955-962.

Ten Hoor, G. A., G. Kok, G. M. Rutten, R. A. Ruiter, S. P. Kremers, A. M. Schols, and G. Plasqui. 2016. "The Dutch 'Focus on Strength' intervention study protocol: programme design and production, implementation and evaluation plan." *BMC Public Health 16:*496.

ten Hoor, G. A., E. F. Sleddens, S. P. Kremers, A. M. Schols, G. Kok, and G. Plasqui. 2015. "Aerobic and strength exercises for youngsters aged 12 to 15: what do parents think?" *BMC Public Health 15:*994.

Thomas, D. M., C. Bouchard, T. Church, C. Slentz, W. E. Kraus, L. M. Redman et al. 2012. "Why do individuals not lose more weight from an exercise intervention at a defined dose? An energy balance analysis." *Obes Rev 13:* 835-847.

Tomkinson, G. R., J. J. Lang, and M. S. Tremblay. 2019. "Temporal trends in the cardiorespiratory fitness of children and adolescents representing 10 high-income and upper middle-income countries between 1981 and 2014." *Br J Sports Med 53(8):*478-486.

Trapp, E. G., D. J. Chisholm, J. Freund, and S. H. Boutcher. 2008. "The effects of high-intensity intermittent exercise training on fat loss and fasting insulin levels of young women." *Int J Obes (Lond) 32 (4):*684-691.

Tremblay, M. S., J. D. Barnes, S. A. González, P. T. Katzmarzyk, V. O. Onywera, J. J. Reilly, G. R. Tomkinson, and Global Matrix 2.0 Research Team. 2016. "Global Matrix 2.0: Report Card Grades on the Physical Activity of Children and Youth Comparing 38 Countries." *J Phys Act Health 13 (11 Suppl 2):*S343-S366.

Umer A., G. A. Kelley, L. E. Cottrell, P. Jr. Giaccobbi, K. E. Innes, C. L. Lilly. 2017. "Childhood obesity and adult cardiovascular disease risk factors: A systematic review with meta-analysis. *BMC Public Health 17(1):*683.

U.S. Department of Health and Human Services. 2018. *Physical activity guidelines for Americans. 2nd edition.* http://www.health.gov/paguidelines/guidelines/.

van Sluijs, E. M., and A. McMinn. 2010. "Preventing obesity in primary schoolchildren." *BMJ 340:*c819.

van Sluijs, E. M., A. M. McMinn, and S. J. Griffin. 2007. "Effectiveness of interventions to promote physical activity in children and adolescents: systematic review of controlled trials." *BMJ 335 (7622):*703.

Vedul-Kjelsås, V., H. Sigmundsson, A. K. Stensdotter, and M. Haga. 2012. "The relationship between motor competence, physical fitness and self-perception in children." *Child Care Health Dev 38 (3):*394-402.

Verstraete, S. J., G. M. Cardon, D. L. De Clercq, and I. M. De Bourdeaudhuij. 2007. "A comprehensive physical activity promotion programme at elementary school: the effects on physical activity, physical fitness and psychosocial correlates of physical activity." *Public Health Nutr 10 (5):*477-484.

Wang, Y., and T. Lobstein. 2006. "Worldwide trends in childhood overweight and obesity." *Int J Pediatr Obes 1 (1):*11-25.

Wareham, N. J., E. M. van Sluijs, and U. Ekelund. 2005. "Physical activity and obesity prevention: a review of the current evidence." *Proc Nutr Soc 64 (2):*229-247.

Weintraub, D. L., E. C. Tirumalai, K. F. Haydel, M. Fujimoto, J. E. Fulton, and T. N. Robinson. 2008. "Team sports for overweight children: the Stanford Sports to Prevent Obesity Randomized Trial (SPORT)." *Arch Pediatr Adolesc Med 162 (3):232-237.*

Weinheimer, E. M., L P. Sands, W. W. Campbell. 2010. "A systematic review of the separate and combined effects of energy restriction and exercise on fat-free mass in middle-aged and older adults: implications for sarcopenic obesity." *Nutr Rev 68:* 375-388.

Westerterp, K. R. 2001. "Pattern and intensity of physical activity." *Nature 410 (6828):*539.

Westerterp, K. R. 2010. "Physical activity, food intake, and body weight regulation: insights from doubly labeled water studies." *Nutr Rev 68 (3):*148-154.

Williams, H. G., K. A. Pfeiffer, J. R. O'Neill, M. Dowda, K. L. McIver, W. H. Brown, and R. R. Pate. 2008. "Motor skill performance and physical activity in preschool children." *Obesity (Silver Spring) 16 (6):*1421-1426.

World, Health Organisation. 2018. *Global action plan on physical activity 2018-2030: more active people for a healthier world.* Geneva, Switzerland: WHO Press.

World Health Organization, World. 2010. *Global recommendations on physical activity for health.* Geneva, Switzerland: WHO Press.

Yanovski, J. A., S. Z. Yanovski, K. N. Sovik, T. T. Nguyen, P. M. O'Neil, and N. G. Sebring. 2000. "A prospective study of holiday weight gain." *N Engl J Med 342 (12):*861-867.

In: Physical Fitness and Exercise
Editor: Quinzia Trevisano

ISBN: 978-1-53618-521-8
© 2020 Nova Science Publishers, Inc.

Chapter 2

AGING PHYSIOLOGY AND PHYSICAL ACTIVITY PRESCRIPTION FOR ELDERLY

Eduardo Borba Neves[1,*],
Gabrielle Cristine Moura Fernandes Pucci[2]
and Francisco Jose Félix Saavedra[3]

[1]Brazilian Army Sports Commission, CDE, Rio de Janeiro, Brazil
and Universidade Tecnológica Federal do Paraná
UTFPR, Curitiba, Brazil
[2]Universidade de Trás-os-Montes e Altos Douro,
UTAD, Vila Real, Portugal
[3]Research Center in Sports Sciences, Health Sciences and
Human Development, CIDESD, Portugal, and Universidade de Trás-os-Montes e Altos Douro, UTAD, Vila Real Portugal

ABSTRACT

This chapter presents the aging physiology and concepts for physical activity prescription for the elderly. To this end, the following topics will

---

* Corresponding Author's E-mail: neveseb@gmail.com.

be discussed: population aging and its challenges; stages and types of aging; physiology of aging (anthropometric changes, cardiac system, respiratory system, nervous system, musculoskeletal system, immune system, and endocrine system); prescription of physical activity for the elderly (concept of physical fitness, muscle strength/endurance training, flexibility training, balance training, cardiorespiratory or aerobic training); and some final considerations. Exercises should be aimed at facilitating the daily lives of the elderly, aiming to work on the needed physical skills for maintaining the autonomy and independence of this population. In this sense, functional activities should be prioritized, thinking about the basic movements that the elderly perform most in their daily lives, such as, for example, walking, getting up from a chair, showering, getting dressed, putting on a shoe.

Keywords: aging, physical training, elderly, physiology

INTRODUCTION

Pontes et al. (2009) define "population aging" or "demographic aging" as the progressive accumulation of larger population groups in the most advanced age groups. Characterized by the reduction in the relative participation of children and young people, accompanied by the proportional increase in adults, especially the elderly in the population.

The elderly population is the fastest-growing worldwide, reflecting the demographic transition, which is a result of the fall in mortality and fertility rates ((WHO) 2002). The demographic transition causes changes in the age structure of the population and is characterized by the transition from a regime with high rates of mortality and fertility to another regime in which there is a reduction to relatively low levels of both rates ((IBGE) 2015).

According to Lebrão (2007), countries can be divided into three groups according to their demographic transition: those with early initiation (European countries), those with late initiation (Latin America and the Caribbean), and those that have not yet begun their transition. (African countries). Aging in developing countries began to be noticed in the mid-twentieth century and occurs in a disordered and very accelerated manner, unlike what happened in developed countries. In developed countries, this demographic transition took place from the 18th century along with the industrial revolution, which resulted in the modernization of European society with advances in different areas. This transition took place gradually, with the population having time and resources to get rich and only later to age. France, for example, took 115 years to increase its elderly population from 7 to 14%, while China will take 27 years to achieve the same increase and Brazil only 19 years ((WHO) 2002, Carvalho 2003, FELIX 2007).

According to the WHO, the last ten years of an elderly person's life are associated with diseases, limitations, and dependencies of some type of special care. To estimate healthy longevity, WHO introduced the concept of healthy life expectancy, which is the number of years of life that are expected to be healthy. This involves disability-adjusted life expectancy (DALE), this calculation takes into account the years of poor health subtracted from the expected overall life expectancy to calculate the equivalent years of healthy life (Mathers 2000).

Given this scenario, QOL longevity is a major challenge for health professionals who must focus their efforts to maintain and/or improve the health of the elderly for as long as possible, with vitality and not longevity being the main focus. WHO stresses that: "It is necessary to recognize that increasing longevity without quality of life is an empty prize. Health expectation is more important than life expectancy." In this sense, this chapter presents the aging physiology and concepts for physical activity (PA) prescription for the elderly.

STAGES AND TYPES OF AGING

Currently, medicine differentiates between two types of aging: senescence and senility. Senescence, also defined as normal aging, is the set of organic, morphological, and functional changes that occur as a result of the natural and healthy aging process. There is a physical and mental decline in the body, but this decline occurs slowly and gradually over the years and has a cumulative effect. The basic needs of daily life such as hygiene, mobility, food, and interpersonal relationships are not compromised. In senility or pathological aging, this decline is marked by changes resulting from chronic pathologies that often affect elderly individuals such as diabetes, high blood pressure, and bad lifestyle habits that can lead to functional disabilities, organ failure, and even death (Miguel 2015, Netto 2006). The consequences of a disease combined with the loss of the ability to maintain homeostasis, trigger several symptoms that determine the loss of autonomy and independence of the elderly.

Still, some authors classify the aging process in three categories: primary, secondary, and tertiary aging. Primary aging is normal, universal aging that will happen to all people regardless of external influences. According to Netto (2002), this type of aging is individually and genetically pre-programmed. According to Spirduso (2005), secondary aging refers to pathologies that are not confused with the natural aging process, resulting from the effects of diseases and environmental factors, among other aspects, such as diet and lifestyle, which can cause different ways of age. Although these two types of aging are distinct, they interact strongly, as environmental stress and diseases increase the individual's vulnerability, consequently accelerating the aging process. For Birren and Schroots (Birren 1996), tertiary aging corresponds to the period marked by great physical and mental losses, arising from the cumulative effects of the aging process and the presence of pathologies.

We must consider that the aging process extends well beyond the age of the individual and that people age in their own way and under different contexts. Therefore, aging should be understood in its entirety, which includes chronological, biological, functional, psychological, and social aging (Netto 2006). Chronological aging registers the passage of time, it is marked by the individual's date of birth and its identification is of paramount importance to record and identify parameters that will follow guidance for planning public policies aimed at the elderly.

Biological aging refers to the decline of the organism in general and is marked by the loss of organ functionality. Biological aging may or may not correspond to chronological aging since the interaction of genetic, environmental and lifestyle factors produces great individual variations. Functional aging, on the other hand, is marked by a physical decline of the body, it is the moment when the person begins to have difficulties to perform their basic activities of daily living such as eating, walking, dressing, getting up, sitting, lying down, directly affecting their autonomy and independence.

Psychological aging is characterized by a mental decline, it is when there are cognitive losses related to memory, attention, perception, judgment, reasoning, thinking, and language. In this, one can mention the empty nest syndrome, which is when parents are faced with the departure of their children from home, and the death of a loved one. People do not prepare themselves emotionally for such moments and, when they arrive, they are psychologically shaken, shortening the aging process. Social aging begins when the individual no longer has a perspective on the future and therefore feels excluded from society in general, ceasing to interact with people and isolating themselves from family and friends, which can often lead to depression deep that can even culminate in death. Social aging depends a lot on the culture in which it is inserted, on the current historical moment, and it is also related to the way people see that elderly person and the way that elderly person positions himself and imposes himself in front of society.

People aged 60 years or older in developing countries and 65 years in developed countries are considered elderly ((ONU) 1982). According to the classification of the World Health Organization ((OMS)), aging consists of four stages, which are:

- Middle age - 45 to 59 years, the period when the first signs of aging begin to appear;
- Elderly - 60 to 74 years old, the phase characterized by the presence of physiological and functional changes typical of old age;
- Old - 75 to 90 years old, a period in which the physiological changes are already well installed, often resulting in limitations and diseases; and
- Very old - over 90 years old, they are usually more fragile and need special care.

Physiology of Aging

Physiological and performance measures generally improve rapidly during childhood and reach their peak between late adolescence and the 30 years, when, from then on, they start to decline with age (Mc Ardle 2016). The process is gradual, progressive, and individual and takes place after the age of 40 when the wear and tear of tissues in relation to the repair of the organism becomes evident (Shepard 2003). During the aging process, the body undergoes a series of physiological changes that gradually decrease the functionality and reserves of our organs and systems. This decline in bodily functions affects several systems such as cardiac, pulmonary, nervous, musculoskeletal and immune systems. However, the speed and extent of these losses vary between systems and also between individuals, since aging does not follow a strict timing in each person and varies according to genetic factors, lifestyle, and environment (Robergs 2002).

Knowledge about the physiology of aging is of fundamental importance to control risk factors and act more safely and effectively in the interventions necessary to improve the QOL of this population.

Anthropometric Modifications

The aging phenotype is represented by typical markers such as gray hair, wrinkled skin, enlargement of the skull cavity, there is also an increase in the size of the nose and ears which gives rise to the facial configuration characteristic of the elderly (Filho 2007).

From the age of 40, the first typical signs of aging begin to manifest, there is a decrease in body height, about 1 cm per decade, this is due to the decrease in plantar arches, arching of the lower limbs, increase the curvatures of the spine and the greater compression of the intervertebral discs, which decrease their water absorption capacity and become more dry and flattened (Filho 2007). This process seems to be more accelerated in women than in men, mainly because of the higher prevalence of osteoporosis after menopause (Matsudo 2000). There is also a reduction in the tricipital and subscapular skinfolds, an increase in the transverse diameter of the chest, also known as the senile chest, and an increase in the anteroposterior diameter of the abdomen (biliary abdomen) (Filho 2007).

Also from 40 years of age, changes in body composition (BC) and body shape begin to manifest, which continues to change progressively until death. The term BC refers to the fractionation of body weight and is divided into four components: fat, bones, muscles, and waste (water, minerals) (Heymsfield 2005). However, for the evaluation of the physical fitness (PF) two components are analyzed: fat mass (FM) and fat free mass (FFM). FFM refers to the part of bodyweight free of fat, is formed by water, muscular and skeletal tissues, skin, organs, and all non-fat tissues (Guedes 1995). The importance of BC focused on PF related to health, is in monitoring the amount of body fat. Evidence points to excess fat as an important risk factor for cardiovascular disease, hypertension, hyperlipidemia, and diabetes, regardless of body weight (ABESO 2009/ 2010, de Koning 2007, Silva 2014). The form of fat distribution is also an important factor since intra-abdominal concentration is a potential risk factor regardless of total body fat (ABESO 2009/ 2010). Just as important as excess body weight, made up of fat, is your deficit. Low body weight can also induce the body to serious complications, with regard to the production and transformation of energy for the maintenance of vital conditions and for the performance of daily activities (ABESO 2009/ 2010).

Among the changes related to BC, there is an increase in body weight, especially between 40 and 60 years, with a subsequent decrease after 70 years (Matsudo 2000). This process is also accompanied by a progressive and continuous loss of skeletal muscle mass, which ends up being largely replaced by fat, most people accumulate 5 to 10 kg of body fat throughout adult life (Shepard 2003). Evidence points that there is an increase of 2 to 5% of body fat per decade and there is a redistribution of adipose tissue that is more concentrated in the central region of the body (visceral fat), accumulating in the trunk and visceral tissues. This type of fat is highly related to the development of cardiovascular diseases, diabetes, dyslipidemia, metabolic syndrome, and some types of cancer (Jansen 2002).

Despite the increase in body fat, there is a reduction in total body weight, this can be explained by the fact that with aging the skeleton becomes demineralized and porous, at the same time, lean body weight tends to decrease with old age (Mc Ardle 2016). For Matsudo et al. (2000) weight loss is multifactorial and is related to changes in neurotransmitters and hormonal factors responsible for controlling hunger and satiety, functional dependence on daily activities related to nutrition, excessive use of medications, depression, financial stress, changes in teething, alcoholism, extreme inactivity, muscle atrophy and catabolism associated with certain diseases. These changes in weight and height consequently also cause changes in the body mass index (BMI) of the elderly.

The body mass index (BMI), despite being a good indicator, cannot be fully correlated with body fat, as it does not distinguish between FFM and FM and may be underestimated in the elderly due to the loss of FFM. In addition, the BMI does not determine how the distribution of body fat occurs (ABESO 2009/2010). Despite these limitations, BMI is more related to weight than height, which is why it has been used for years and on a large scale as a general indication of healthy weight management.

Cardiovascular System

Risk factors for the development of cardiovascular diseases are more prevalent and severe with advancing age (Costa 2015). Statistics show that ischemic heart disease is the main cause of mortality in Brazil among elderly people over 70 years of age, but due to the high incidence of cardiac and vascular diseases that affect the elderly, there is a great difficulty in recognizing which changes result specifically from the aging process (Affiune 2006).

With advancing age, the heart and blood vessels show morphological and tissue changes even in the absence of any disease, and the set of these changes has become known as the senile heart (Affiune 2006). The changes in the myocardium are the most significant, there is an increase in thickness and accumulation of fat in the walls of the atria, ventricles, and interventricular septum (Costa 2015, Shepard 2003).

With aging, there is a progressive decrease in the maximum heart rate of about 1 bpm per year, but the resting heart rate is not affected by any relevant modification (Spirduso 2005). The decrease in maximum heart rate seems to occur to the same degree in both active and sedentary men and women (Mc Ardle 2016). In response to this lower peak heart rate, there is a reduction in maximum cardiac output (Booth 1994). A reduced cardiac ejection volume also contributes to this reduced cardiac flow capacity, which can result from changes in myocardial contractility (Mc Ardle 2016). The greatest changes in heart rate are observed during submaximal and maximum exercises since the lowest peak heart rate and the attenuated contractile responses of the left ventricle reduce maximum cardiac output, maximum oxygen consumption, and the ability to exercise. The elderly person will not reach the maximum heart rate when he was younger due to less loss of cardiac vagal tone and the fact that the heart is less sensitive to beta-adrenergic stimulations (Seals 1994).

The capacity of the venous system is increased by a progressive reduction in venous tone and the development of numerous varicosities. There is also cholesterol, impaired cardiac conduction, and reduced baroreceptor function, in addition to degeneration, calcification, and decreased distensibility of the aorta and large arteries. Over the years, blood vessels become more resistant and suffer a progressive loss of elasticity in the great arteries, leading to an increase in blood pressure during rest and exercise, an alteration in the pulse wave in the blood and an increase in pressure against which ventricle should be emptied (Affiune 2006, Costa 2015). This greater rigidity in the arterial walls is known as arteriosclerosis, which is a condition caused by the formation of fibrous tissues and progressive calcification of the arteries (Shepard 2003).

It is not yet known whether changes in cardiovascular function are exclusive to the aging process itself or whether it is the result of the absence of regular physical activity. In fact, sedentary living can cause losses in functional capacity as significant as the deleterious effects of aging. Training studies suggest that regular physical exercise allows elderly individuals to perform cardiovascular conditioning much higher than sedentary individuals of an equivalent age (Mc Ardle 2016).

Respiratory System

With aging, structural and functional changes are observed that lead to a progressive decline in the respiratory system. These changes are characterized by a set of physiological changes that affect the lungs, rib cage, and respiratory muscles, causing impairment in lung function that varies in amplitude between individuals and that are dependent on endogenous and exogenous factors (Gorzoni 2006).

Among these changes, we can mention the changes in the chest morphology, which determine the configuration of the senile chest, the reduction of elasticity and the atrophy of the skeletal muscles associated with breathing, as a result of these changes, the capacity of expansion of the rib cage is reduced (Filho 2007). Other changes are weakening of the respiratory muscles, loss of lung retraction, reduced chest compliance, increased lung compliance, increased residual volume, reduced vital capacity, reduced inspiratory capacity, reduced forced expiratory volume, increased ventilation during exercise, and decreased pulmonary diffusion capacity (Shepard 2003).

The elderly also have a lower consumption of VO2 max which, together with the reduction in the strength of the respiratory muscles, leads to a lesser capacity to sustain muscle resistance exercises and requires a longer recovery time between one exercise and another, which may affect physical conditioning (Netto 2006).

Nervous System

The nervous system is responsible for coordinating and regulating most of the control functions of our organism. Safons and Balsamo (2005) cite the central nervous system (CNS) as the system most compromised by aging, because, in addition to the internal biological functions, it is the system responsible for movements, sensations, and psychic functions, not to mention that it has no reparative capacity and additionally it is influenced by intrinsic and extrinsic factors.

The changes associated with the aging of this system are a decrease of approximately 40% in the number of medullary axons, a decrease in dendrites, neurons and the number of synapses at the cortical level, changes in sensitivity, changes in neurotransmitters with slowing of complex mental functions, reduction strength and idle speed (Filho 2007). There is also a decrease in muscle excitability and nerve conduction speed with an impaired motor response to stimuli, decreasing the intensity of reflexes and consequently delaying reaction and movement time, from the simplest to the most complex (Mc Ardle 2016). These modifications, together with changes in autonomic systemic function, which causes variations in blood pressure with the risk of orthostatic hypotension, can cause serious impairments in the health of the elderly, being responsible for a greater number of falls and injuries that can generate fractures and even death (Aguiar 2006).

Musculoskeletal System

The musculoskeletal system is one of the systems most affected by aging and one of the most impacting on the QOL of the elderly, as it is directly related to locomotion, postural support, and the ability to generate movements and perform daily activities (Pucci 2016).

Changes in the muscular system include an increase in the size of non-contractile tissue in the muscle, a reduction in the cross-sectional area, a reduction in the number and size of fibers, mainly type II, atrophy of muscle fibers, there is also a progressive loss of alpha motor neurons with reduction of motor units (Doherty 2003). All of these changes result in a reduction in muscle strength and volume, which occurs with greater intensity in the lower limbs (Goodpaster 2006, Hughes 2001).

Muscle strength (MS) begins to decline around age 40, accelerating after age 60. For every decade, after the age of 25, 3% to 5% of FFM is lost

(Robergs 2002), due to the losses in bone mass, skeletal muscle, and total body water that happen during aging (Matsudo 2000). Although FFM is composed of water, viscera, bone, connective tissue, and muscle, muscle is the one that most suffers loss with the aging process, around 40%. The main causes of this selective loss are the decrease in the levels of growth hormone and the increase in physical inactivity that happens with advancing age (Matsudo 2000).

It is agreed that the biggest deficit from the functional point of view for the elderly is the reduction of MS because it generates a series of implications that can compromise the health, quality of life and activities of daily living of the elderly, making even simple activities and routines such as walking, bathing, cleaning the house, getting up and sitting on a chair, require a great physical effort (Fleck 2017). In view of this greater difficulty in performing routine activities, the elderly tend to become less and less active, resulting in weaker muscles and atrophied by disuse, further aggravating the loss of FFM through a vicious cycle (Nóbrega et al. 1999). Consequently to the loss of FFM, there is a reduction in strength, this characteristic phenomenon of aging is known as sarcopenia. Rosenberg (2011) defines sarcopenia as the involuntary loss of muscle mass and function associated with old age, being a disease that can be diagnosed and treated. The causes for sarcopenia are multiple and are related to mitochondrial dysfunction, decreased size and death of muscle fibers, weakening of the contractile potential of actin and myosin, endocrine changes, nutritional disorders, physical inactivity, immobility and neurodegenerative diseases (Esquenazi 2014, Perfeito 2014).

Another process inherent to aging are postural changes, due to muscle weakness, the elderly tend to assume incorrect and compensatory postures. In addition to the postural decrease mentioned above, there is an increase in the angle of the knees due to the shortening of the hamstring muscles, this shortening ends up causing a pelvic retroversion, thus decreasing lumbar lordosis. In addition, the antigravity muscles and the anterior and posterior ligaments that support the spine are losing strength and decreasing their function of supporting the posture, contributing to the adoption of the forward flexed posture, which modifies the center of gravity compromising the balance and making the elderly more susceptible to falls and fractures (Esquenazi 2014).

With advancing age the bones become more fragile and porous. As the bone loses calcium it becomes more vulnerable to fractures. This loss of calcium results in a decrease in bone mass, which is more pronounced among women, especially after menopause. After the age of 50, men tend to decrease about 1% of bone mass per year, while women begin to lose it by age 30, with a drop of 2 to 3% per year after menopause. Bone mass among men decreases approximately 10% up to 65 years and about 20% up to 80 years. Among women, the loss is approximately 20% at 65 years old and 30% at 80 years old (Robergs 2002).

Immune System

The term immunosenescence refers to immune aging that is associated with a progressive decline in immune function and that contributes to a higher incidence of infectious, chronic-degenerative, autoimmune, and neoplastic diseases after 60 years of age (Tonet 2008). Among the changes that occur in this system can be mentioned: involution and atrophy of the thymus, which gradually up to 50 years of age, loses up to 95% of its mass and capacity to produce hormones; decreased cellular immunity, mainly the ability of suppressor T cells to recognize and eliminate antigens in relation to the body's own (Filho 2007); and defects in lineage B leading to a greater encounter of antibodies, greater susceptibility to infectious diseases, reactivations of latent infections and the appearance of neoplasms (Aguiar 2006).

Although old age is not necessarily linked to diseases and disabilities, the changes resulting from aging contribute to a greater vulnerability of these individuals to adverse health manifestations. The diseases that most affect the elderly can be classified as neurodegenerative (Alzheimer's, Parkinson's), cardiodegenerative (coronary artery disease, heart failure, stroke, hypertension, type II diabetes mellitus), osteodegenerative (osteoporosis, osteoarthrosis, spinal pain, and chronic pain) and others such as cancer, bronchitis, depression, circulatory disorders, and metabolic disorders.

The most common chronic non-communicable diseases in old age are Systemic Arterial Hypertension, followed by Diabetes Mellitus, which together are considered the main risk factors for the development of kidney complications, heart and cerebrovascular diseases (Duncan 2012).

Endocrine System

The endocrine system substantially loses its ability to measure the endogenous hormonal dosage, causing some hormones to lose the function of satisfactorily responding to the exercise stimulus, as in the case of testosterone and growth hormone (GH), which are essential for maintaining and gaining weight. strength (Perfeito 2014). After a strength training session, serum concentrations of anabolic hormones increase above resting values during and after the training session, thereby stimulating muscle remodeling and growth (Fleck 2017). However, with aging, the endocrine system loses its ability to alter hormonal concentrations caused by exercise, reductions in resting concentrations of anabolic hormones are also observed (Fleck 2017).

PRESCRIPTION OF PHYSICAL ACTIVITY FOR ELDERLY

The Sedentary lifestyle leads to losses in functional capacity at least as significant as old age itself. Although exercise is not able to interrupt the aging process, there is sufficient evidence pointing to the inverse relationship between physical exercise and some types of diseases (Katzmarzyk 2004, Fransson 2004, Committee. 2008). Regular physical exercise is able to improve physiological function at any age, however, initial physical fitness, genetics, type, and amount of training control the magnitude of these changes (Mc Ardle 2016).

The realization of an efficient and well-targeted exercise program works to prevent and rehabilitate the health of the elderly and should aim to improve physical fitness and functional capacity. Matsudo (2000) describes a physical activity program that includes aerobic training, strength training, and specific balance and flexibility exercises as the best exercise option for the elderly. For Jacob Filho (2006), a balanced program should include muscle strengthening, balance and coordination exercises, aiming to improve the gait pattern, reflexes and thus reduce the incidence of falls in the elderly.

Concept of Physical Fitness

Physical fitness (PF) is defined as the physical ability to perform daily activities in a safe and autonomous manner without excessive fatigue (Guedes 1995). For the American College of Sports Medicine (2010), we can understand PF as a "series of attributes that people have or acquire and that relate to the ability to perform physical activity." According to Böhme (2003), PF is a set of multiple characteristics that extends from birth to death and must be developed during all stages of life. Given these definitions, it is understood that maintaining good physical fitness is a crucial factor throughout life to have good health and have a functional capacity satisfactory to the demands of everyday life.

The components of the PF encompass different dimensions and can have two aspects, one focused on health and the other on sports performance (Araújo 2000). The components related to health are those components that are directly proportional to the best health status and include the variables of strength, flexibility, maximum aerobic power, and components of body composition. While the PF focused on sports performance includes the variables of agility, balance, motor coordination, power, and speed (Guedes 1995). In this study, in addition to the PF parameters related to health, we also chose to include balance assessment, as it is a very important variable for the elderly since it undergoes major changes over the years and is a fundamental requirement for independent aging. Corroborating this idea,

Morrow (2003) states that the PF of an elderly person should include factors of motor aptitude, such as balance, reaction time, and movement time in order to maintain functional capacity, activities of daily living, and global QOL.

ACSM and AHA ((ACSM) 2009a, Services. 2008, Leavitt 2008) developed the current recommendations for physical exercise for the elderly. These recommendations were based on epidemiological studies with worldwide coverage and extensive scientific evidence. The purpose of these recommendations is to minimize public health problems caused by physical inactivity and to ensure that the elderly obtain maximum health benefits through exercise. The current recommendations recommend that in order to have good health and avoid chronic-degenerative diseases, the elderly must perform aerobic activities, strength exercises, flexibility, and balance at least twice a week.

Strength Training/Resistance Training

Muscle strength (MS) and endurance are vital factors for health, functional capacity, and performance of activities of daily living. Strength is understood as the neuromuscular ability to win, oppose, or sustain resistance that can be used by external loads or by supporting one's own body weight (Perfeito 2014). While muscle resistance is the ability of muscles to exert submaximal strength repeatedly over a period of time (Moreira 2001). With aging, there is a loss of muscle strength and resistance resulting mainly from the process of loss of FFM, a decrease in the level of PF, and an increase in the percentage of fat (Toss 2012, Lustgarten 2011). Muscle weakness can be a very limiting factor in the independence of the elderly, preventing them from performing common activities such as housework, descending and climbing stairs, rising from a chair, among many others.

The regular practice of strength training is associated with a reduced risk of morbidity and mortality in the elderly (Drenowatz 2015, Kraschnewski 2016), as well as with better walking speed and reduced risk of falls (Cadore 2013, Santos 2017). Maintaining MS should be the highest priority for working with the elderly. It is important to include strength training for the elderly, especially for the lower limbs (lower limbs), which seem to be the most affected with aging. The reduction in the strength of the lower limbs is predictive of the onset of physical disability at older ages (Rikli 2008).

In addition to the loss of strength, there is also a decrease in muscle power, which is the muscle's ability to develop strength quickly. The preservation of muscle strength and power are protective mechanisms for falls, which represent a major public health problem, and one of the most important causes of injuries and fractures in the elderly (Fleck 2017).

Studies show that strength training can be successfully and safely implemented in the elderly, including among the sick and frail. Research has shown that regular resistance training is able to recover much of the lost strength and FFM resulting in improved functional mobility. According to the American College of Sports Medicine (ACSM), strength is one of the most important variables for the functioning of the body, and strength training is the main activity to achieve high levels of PF related to health and should be stimulated in all areas. age groups ((ACSM) 2009b).

Strength training comprises all the action that aims to maximize, recover, or maintain already existing strength levels (Perfeito 2014). In order to maintain and improve muscle strength / endurance levels, it is necessary to exercise regularly at levels more intense than required in daily life. For this, one can use the overload of one's own body weight or make use of exercises that use an external overload, such as loaded devices, dumbbells, ribbons, elastic bands, etc. (Guedes 1995).

As for strength exercises for elderly beginners, the intensity should be light, varying between 40-50% of 1 repetition maximum (RM), progressing later to moderate intensity of 60 to 70% of 1 RM. The exercise program should be performed on a frequency of 2 to 3 times a week, lasting approximately 30 minutes each session and should include progressive exercises that involve large muscle groups. The exercises can be carried out with the support of their own body weight, with free weights or with loaded devices.

As the preservation of MS is vital during the aging process, its measurement assumes a crucial role to evaluate the PF and to develop PF programs focused on the health of the elderly (Rikli 2008).

Flexibility Training

As you get older the joints become less flexible and more rigid, compromising the good performance of the locomotor system. Changes in the connective tissue of muscles, ligaments, joint capsules, and tendons are one of the factors responsible for the loss of flexibility and mobility in the elderly (Moreira 2001). For Almeida (2009), the limitations in the range of motion are the result of an increase in the proportion of connective tissue in FFM, dehydration of the joint and a change in the composition of elastin and collagen that undergoes a reduction in the length of the chondroitin chains in the articular cartilage. Collagen cells are important structures that contribute to maintaining the integrity of joint components, however, over time, collagen undergoes progressive degeneration (Esquenazi 2014).

According to Dantas (1999), flexibility is a "physical quality responsible for the voluntary execution of a movement of maximum angular amplitude, for a joint or set of joints, within the morphological limits, without the risk of causing injury." Flexibility is an important physical quality for the good performance of the usual activities of the elderly, such as putting on a shoe, dressing, bathing, reaching for an object. The loss of this valence restricts the range of movements and can seriously compromise the mobility of the elderly. Dantas (2001) points out that a range of articulation capable of generating conditions for the good execution of daily movements contributes to the elderly being able to maintain their independence and have a greater willingness to face the challenges of daily life.

Considering that the flexibility of a joint depends on its level of use, disuse can contribute to a decrease in the range of motion of the joints, favoring the functional limitation of the elderly (Dantas 2001). To maintain and increase muscle stability and flexibility levels, the literature recommends stretching exercises. Flexibility exercises should be performed

2-3 times a week, with moderate intensity ranging from 5-6 points using the Borg scale adapted from 0 to 10, where 0 represents the minimum effort and 10 the maximum effort. The movements must be static, capable of maintaining or increasing flexibility through sustained and slow stretches for the main muscle groups. The time in the position for each exercise should vary from 30-60 seconds.

For Cyrino et al. (2004), involvement in regular physical exercise programs, regardless of the practice of specific flexibility exercises, can be a good strategy to improve levels of flexibility, especially among sedentary people, since the joints that are not used often will begin to receive a new progressive stimulus that will cause positive adaptations in the medium or long term (Cyrino 2004). Guedes (1995) argues that elderly people who have better levels of flexibility tend to move more easily and are less susceptible to injuries when subjected to more intense physical efforts.

Balance Training

Balance is a vital factor for human beings because without it it would be difficult or even impossible to perform tasks such as walking, standing, jumping, turning, among others. Balance can be described as the ability to control the position of the body in space for purposes of support and orientation (Granacher 2012) and comes in three forms: proactive balance (anticipation of a predicted disturbance), static / dynamic balance (maintaining a position stable, stopped or in motion) and reactive balance (ability to recover the balance from any position) (Shumway-Cook A.; Woollacott 2007).

Maintaining body balance requires the interaction of the vestibular, somatosensory, and visual systems. The vestibular system perceives linear and angular accelerations, the somatosensory is sensitive to the position and speed of all body segments and the visual system captures the colors, shapes, and movements of objects and the body itself (Mann 2008). The aging process compromises the ability of the central nervous system to perform the processing of vestibular, visual, and proprioceptive signals, in addition to decreasing the ability to modify adaptive reflexes. These degenerative processes are responsible for postural instability (Ruwer 2005).

In addition to changes in the biological system, postural changes that occur with aging can influence the maintenance of body balance. The lack of balance has a great impact on the lives of the elderly, which can impair the performance of daily activities and lead to social isolation, in addition to contributing to the increase in public spending resulting from high rates of falls and fractures (Mann 2008). The practice of specific physical exercises for balance increases self-confidence (Spirduso 2005) and is seen as a strong tool to improve balance, decrease the risk of falls and fractures in the elderly.

There is insufficient evidence as to the frequency, intensity, type, and time of balance training, however, it is suggested that the combination of balance, agility, and proprioceptive exercises are effective in preventing and reducing the incidence of falls when performed at least twice in the week. Exercises must include dynamic movements that disturb the center of gravity, postures that become progressively more difficult, and reduced support, just as in other valences, large muscle groups should be prioritized.

Cardiorespiratory or Aerobic Training

Cardiorespiratory fitness is defined by the body's ability to adapt to moderate physical efforts, involving large muscle groups, for relatively long periods of time (Guedes 1995). The cardiorespiratory function requires intense participation of the respiratory and cardiovascular systems, which has the function of delivering oxygen to tissues while removing carbon dioxide (Moreira 2001). When a person is subjected to a physical effort, the active muscles require increasing amounts of oxygen in order to produce the energy necessary to meet the required effort. Therefore, people who have a higher level of aerobic capacity tend to have greater ease and efficiency in performing daily activities, in addition to recovering more quickly after performing more intense physical efforts (Guedes 1995).

A sedentary lifestyle can contribute to poor cardiorespiratory performance, progressively decreasing the individual's ability to perform the physical effort. Maintaining an adequate level of aerobic activity has a direct effect on functional mobility and indirectly on reducing the risk of illness (Rikli 2008). Aerobic endurance is necessary for several daily activities such as walking, climbing and descending stairs, shopping, and participating in recreational and sports activities. The assessment of cardiorespiratory fitness measures the ability to participate in activities considered normal, as well as the physiological reserves necessary to participate in physical activities considered at a pleasant pace (Moreira 2001).

In relation to aerobic activities, the recommendation is to practice 75-150 min per week of aerobic activity with vigorous-intensity or 150-300 min per week of moderate aerobic activity. The authors emphasize that when the elderly are unable to reach the recommended levels because of some limitation or chronic condition, they should remain as physically active as their condition allows. The ACSM (2010) also recommends that, in order to obtain more health benefits, the elderly should whenever possible exceed the recommended minimum values.

CONCLUSION

It is of utmost importance that professionals develop a physical exercise program aiming to meet not only the needs but also seeking the acceptance and satisfaction of those who will practice it, in order to avoid disinterest and abandonment of the activity. The exercises should be aimed at facilitating the daily life of the elderly, aiming to work on the aforementioned skills with the main objective of maintaining the autonomy and independence of this population. In this sense, functional activities should be prioritized, thinking about the basic movements that the elderly perform most in their daily lives, such as walking, getting up from a chair, showering, getting dressed, putting on a shoe. Therefore, it is essential that professionals are qualified to work with this population and that they know the changes resulting from aging, so that they can act safely and effectively, proposing exercises that meet the biological needs of the elderly, in order to mitigate the effects deleterious effects of aging.

REFERENCES

ACSM, American College of Sports Medicine. 2009a. Exercise Activity for Older Adults. *Official Journal of the American College of Sports Medicine.*

ACSM, American College of Sports Medicine. 2009b. Progression models in resistance training for healthy adults. *Med Sci Sports Exerc.* 41 (3):687-708.

ACSM, American College of Sports Medicine. 2010. *ACSM's Guidelines for Exercising Testing and Prescription.* Philadelphia: Lippincot Williams & Wilkins.

IBGE, Instituto Brasileiro de Geografia e Estatística. 2015. *Mudança Demográfica no Brasil no Início do Século XXI.* accessed 08/10/2018. [*Demographic Change in Brazil at the Beginning of the 21st Century.*]

OMS, Organização Mundial Saúde. (ONU), ORGANIZAÇÃO DAS NAÇÕES UNIDAS. 1982. *Assembléia mundial sobre envelhecimento: resolução 39/125.* Viena. [*World Assembly on Aging: Resolution 39/125.*]

WHO, World Health Organization. 2002. *Active Ageing: A Policy Framework.* Second United Nations World Assembly on Ageing, Madrid, Spain.

ABESO. 2009/ 2010. Diretrizes brasileiras de obesidade. In *Sobrepeso e obseidade: diagnóstico.* São Paulo: AC Farmacêutica. [Brazilian obesity guidelines. In *Overweight and obesity: diagnosis.*]

Affiune, A. 2006. Envelhecimento Cardiovascular. In *Tratado de Geratria e Gerontologia,* edited by E. V.; Py Freitas, L.; Cançado, F. A. X; Doll, J.; Gorzoni, M. L. Rio de Janeiro: Guanabara Koogan. [Cardiovascular aging. In *Treaty of Geriatrics and Gerontology*]

Aguiar, E. 2006. Alterações Laboratoriais no Envelhecimento. In *Geriatria,* edited by L. H. H. Hargreaves. Brasília. [Laboratory Changes in Aging. In *Geriatrics*]

Almeida, T. C. 2009. *Avaliação da aptidão física de idosas do programa de ginástica matinal da cidade de Barretos-SP: uma proposta para a prooção da saúde.* Mestrado, Universidade de Franca. [*Physical fitness assessment of elderly women in the morning gymnastics program in the city of Barretos-SP: a proposal for health promotion.*]

Araújo, D. S. M. S.; Araújo, C. G. S. 2000. Aptidão física, saúde e qualidade de vida relacionada à saúde em adultos. *Rev Bras Med Esporte* 6 (5):194-203. [Physical fitness, health and health-related quality of life in adults. *Rev Bras Med Sport*]

Birren, J. E.; E Schroots, J. J. F., 1996. History, concepts and theory in the psychology of aging. In *Handook of The Psychologu of aging 4 ed.*, edited by J. E.; Schaie Birren, K. W., 3-23. San Diego: Academic Press.

Bohme, M. T. S. 2003. Relações entre aptidão física, esporte e treinamento esportivo. *R. bras. Ci. e Mov* 11 (3):97-104. [Relationships between physical fitness, sport and sports training.]

Booth, F. W.; Weeden, S. H.; Tseng, B. S. 1994. Effect of aging on human skeletal muscle and motor function. *Med. Sci. Sports Exerc.* 26:556-560.

Cadore, E. L.; Rodríguez-Manãs, L.; Sinclair, A.; Izquierdo, M. 2013. Effects of different exercise interventions on risk of falls, gait ability, and balance in physically frail older adults: a systematic review. *Rejuvenation Research* 16 (2):105-114.

Carvalho, J. A. M.; Garcia, R. A. 2003. O envelhecimento da população brasileira: um enfoque demográfico. *Cad. Saúde Pública,* 19 (23):725-733. [The aging of the Brazilian population: a demographic approach]

Committee, Physical Activity Guidelines Advisory. 2008. *Physical Activity Guidelines Advisory Committee Report.* Washington, DC: U.S.: US Department of Health and Human Services.

Costa, J. A.; Segheto, W.; Ribeiro, P. V. M.; Milagres, L. C.; Tinôco, E. F.; Rosa, C. O. B.; Tinôco, A. L. A. 2015. Sistema Cardiovascular. In *Saúde do Idoso Epidemiologia, Aspectos Nutricionais e Processo do Envelhecimento*, edited by A. L. A.; Rosa Tinôco, C. O. B. Rio de Janeiro: Rubio. [Cardiovascular system. In *Health of the Elderly Epidemiology, Nutritional Aspects and the Aging Process*]

Cyrino, E. S.; Oliveira, A. R.; Leite, J. C.; Porto, D. B.; Dias, R. M. R.; Segantin, A. Q., et al. 2004. Comportamento da flexibilidade após 10 semanas de treinamento com pesos. *Rev Bras Med Esporte* 10 (4):233-237. [Flexibility behavior after 10 weeks of weight training.]

Dantas, H. M. 1999. *Flexibilidade: alongamento e flexionamento*. Rio de Janeiro: Shape. [*Flexibility: stretching and flexing*]

Dantas, E. H. M.; Costa, D. M.; Pereira, S. A. M. 2001. Flexibilidade na terceira idade. In *Atividade Física na Maturidade*, edited by C. A. Moreira. Rio de Janeiro: Shape. [Flexibility in old age. In *Physical Activity at Maturity*]

de Koning, L.; Merchant, A. T.; Pogue,J.; Anand, S. S. 2007. Waist circumference and waist-to-hip ratio as predictors of cardiovascular events: meta-regression analysis of prospective studies. *Eur Heart J.* 28 (7):850-6.

Doherty, T. J. 2003. Invited Review: Aging and Sarcopenia. *Journal of Applied Physiology* 95:1717-1727.

Drenowatz, C.; Sui, X.; Fritz, S.; Lavie, C. J.; Beatti, P. F.; Church, T. S.; Blair, S. N. 2015. The association between resistance exercise and cardiovascular disease risk in women. *Journal of Science and Medicine in Sport* 18 (6):632-636.

Duncan, B. B.; Chor, D.; Aquino, E. M. L.; Bensenor, I. M.; Mill, J. G.; Schmidt, M. I. 2012. Doenças crônicas não transmissíveis no Brasil: prioridade para enfrentamento e investigação. *Rev Saúde Pública* 46 (1):126-134. [Chronic non-communicable diseases in Brazil: priority for coping and investigation]

Esquenazi, D.; da Silav, S. R. B; Guimarães, M. A. M. 2014. Aspectos fisiopatológicos do envelhecimento humano e quedas em idosos. *Revista HUPE* 13 (2):11-20. [Pathophysiological aspects of human aging and falls in the elderly.]

Felix, J. S. 2007. O planeta dos idosos. *Revista Fator*. [The planet of the elderly. *Fator Magazine*]

Filho, E. T. C. 2007. Fisiologia do Envelhecimento. In *Tratado de Gerontologia*, edited by M. Papaléo Netto. São Paulo: Atheneu. [Physiology of Aging. In *Treaty of Gerontology*]

Fleck, S. J.; Kraemer, W. J., ed. 2017. *Fundamentos do Treinamento de Força Muscular*. Edited by 4 edição. Porto Alegre: Artmed. [*Fundamentals of Muscle Strength Training*]

Fransson, E; Ahlbom, A; Reuterwall, C; Hallqvist, J; Alfredsson, L. 2004. The Risk of Acute Myocardial Infarction: Interactions of Types of Physical Activity. *Epidemiology* 15 (5):573-582.

Goodpaster, B. H.; Park, S. W.; Harris, T. B.; Kritchevsky, S. B.; Nevitt, M.; Schwartz, A. V. et al. 2006. The loss of skeletal muscle strength, mass, and quality in older adults: the health, aging and body composition study. *J Gerontol A Biol Sci Med Sci.* 61 (10):1059-64.

Gorzoni, M. L.; Russo, M. R. 2006. Envelhecimento Respiratório. In *Tratado de Geriatria e Gerontologia*, edited by E. V.; Py Freitas, L.; Cançado, F. A. X; Doll, J.; Gorzoni, M. L. Rio de Janeiro: Guanabara Koogan. [Respiratory aging. In *Treaty of Geriatrics and Gerontology*]

Granacher, U.; Muehlbauer, T.; Gruber, M. 2012. A Qualitative Review of Balance and Strength Performance in Healthy Older Adults: Impact for Testing and Training. *J Aging Res.*: 1-16.

Guedes, D. P.; Guedes, J. E. R. P. 1995. Atividade Física, Aptidão Física e Saúde. *Revista Brasileira de Atividade Física e Saúde* 1 (1):18-35. [Physical Activity, Physical Fitness and Health. *Brazilian Journal of Physical Activity and Health*]

Heymsfield, S. B.; Lohman, T. G.; Wang, J.; Going, S. B. 2005. *Human Body Composition*. Edited by 2 ed.: Human Kinetics.

Hughes, V. A.; Frontera, W. R.; Wood, M.; Evans, W. J.; Dallal, G. E.; Roubenoff, R. et al. 2001. Longitudinal muscle strength changes in older adults: influence of muscle mass, physical activity, and health. *J Gerontol A Biol Sci Med Sci.* 56:209-17.

Jacob Filho, W. 2006. Atividade física e envelhecimento saudável. *Rev. bras. Educ. Fís. Esp.* 20:73-77. [Physical activity and healthy aging]

Jansen, I.; Katzmarzyk, P. T.; Ross, R. 2002. Body mass index, waist circumference, and health risk. *Arch Intern Med* 162 (18):2074-79.

Katzmarzyk, P. T.; Janssen, I. 2004. The economic costs associated with physical inactivity and obesity in Canada: an update. *Canadian Journal of Applied Physiology* 29 (1):90-115.

Kraschnewski, J. L.; Sciamanna, C. N.; Poger, J. M.; Rovniak, L. S.; Lehman, E. B.; Cooper, A. B.; Ballentine, N. H.; Ciccolo, J. T. 2016. Is strength training associated with mortality benefits? A 15 year cohort study of US older adults. *Preventive Medicine* 87:121-127.

Leavitt, M. O. 2008. *Physical Activity Guidelines for Americans*, edited by U.S. Department of Health and Human Services. Washington.

Lebrão, M. L. 2007. O envelhecimento no Brasil: aspectos da transição demográfica e epidemiológica. *Saúde Coletiva* 4 (17):135-140. [Aging in Brazil: aspects of the demographic and epidemiological transition. *Collective Health*]

Lustgarten, M. S.; Fielding, R. A. 2011. Assessment of analytical methods used to measure changes in body composition in the elderly and recommendations for their use in phase ii clinical trials. *The Journal Nutrition Health Aging* 15 (5):368-375.

Mann, L.; Kleinpaula, J. F.; Teixeira, C. S.; Rossi, A. G.; Lopes, L. F. D.; Mota, C. B. 2008. Investigação do equilíbrio corporal em idosos. *Rev. Bras. Geriatr. Gerontol.* 11 (2):155-165. [Investigation of body balance in the elderly]

Mathers, C. D.; Sadana, R.; Salomon, J. A.; Murray, C. J. L.; Lopez, A. D. 2000. Estimates of DALE for 191 countries: methods and results. In *Global Programme on Evidence for Health Policy Working Paper n.16*, edited by World Health Organization.

Matsudo, S. M.; Matsudo, V.; Neto, T. L. B. 2000. Impacto do envelhecimento nas variáveis antropométricas, neuromotoras e metabólicas da aptidão física. *Rev. Bras. Ciên. e Mov.* 8 (4):21-32. [Impact of aging on anthropometric, neuromotor and metabolic variables of physical fitness.]

Mc Ardle, W.; Katch, F. I.; Katch, V. L. 2016. *Fisiologia do exercício: Energia, Nutrição e Desempenho*. Edited by 8 edição, *Editora Guanabara*. Rio de Janeiro. [*Exercise physiology: Energy, Nutrition and Performance*]

Miguel, E. S.; Sediyama, C. M. N. O; Oliveira, M. F.; de Souza, J. D.; Montini,T. A.; Tinôco, A. L. A. 2015. Senescência e Senilidade. In *Saúde do Idoso Epidemiologia, Aspectos Nutricionais e Processos do Envelhecimento*, edited by A. L. A.; Rosa Tinôco, C. O. B. Rio de

Janeiro: Rubio. [Senescence and Senility. In *Health of the Elderly Epidemiology, Nutritional Aspects and Aging Processes*]

Moreira, C. A. 2001. *Atividade Física na Maturidade*. Edited by 1 ed. Rio de Janeiro: Shape. [Physical Activity at Maturity]

Morrow, J. R. 2003. *Medida e avaliação do desempenho humano*. Edited by 2 ed. Porto Alegre: Artmed. [*Measurement and evaluation of human performance*]

Netto, M. P. 2006. O Estudo da Velhice: Histórico, Definição do Campo e Termos Básicos. In *Tratado de Geriatria e Gerontologia*, edited by E. V.; Py Freitas, L.; Cançado, F. A. X; Doll, J.; Gorzoni, M. L. Rio de Janeiro: Guanabara Koogan. [The Study of Old Age: History, Definition of the Field and Basic Terms. In *Treaty of Geriatrics and Gerontology*]

Netto, P. M. 2002. *Gerontologia: a velhice e o envelhecimento em visão globalizada*. Edited by Atheneu. São Paulo. [*Gerontology: old age and aging in a global view*]

Nóbrega, A. C. L., E. V. Freitas, M. A. B. Oliveira, M. B. Leitão, J. K. Lazzoli, R. M. Nahas, C. A. S. Baptista, F. A. Drummond, L. Rezende, and J. Pereira. 1999. Posicionamento oficial da Sociedade Brasileira de Medicina do Esporte e da Sociedade Brasileira de Geriatria e Gerontologia: atividade física e saúde no idoso. *Revista Brasileira de Medicina do Esporte* 5 (6):207-211. [Official positioning of the Brazilian Society of Sports Medicine and the Brazilian Society of Geriatrics and Gerontology: physical activity and health in the elderly. *Brazilian Journal of Sports Medicine*]

Perfeito, R. S. 2014. *Método Pilates uma possível intervençao para a promoção da saúde no envelhecimento, 1 ed*. Rio de Janeiro: Kirios. [*Pilates Method a possible intervention for the promotion of health in aging, 1st ed*]

Pontes, R. J. S.; Júnior, A. N. R.; Kerr, L. R. S.; Bosi, M. L. M. 2009. Transição Demográfica e Epidemiológica. In *Epidemiologia*, edited by Roberto de Andrade Medronho. São Paulo: Atheneu. [Demographic and Epidemiological Transition. In *Epidemiology*]

Pucci, G.; Sarabia, T. T. 2016. Pilates e envelhecimento. In *Pilates 360*, edited by T. A. Costa. Erechim: Deviant. [Pilates and aging. In *Pilates 360*]

Rikli, R. E.; Jones, C. J. 2008. *Teste de Aptidão Física para Idosos*. Edited by 1 ed. São Paulo: Manole. [*Physical Fitness Test for the Elderly*]

Robergs, R. A.; Roberts, S. O. 2002. *Fisiologia do Exercício para Aptidão, Desesmpenho e Saúde*. Edited by 1 ediçào, *Phorte Editora*. São Paulo. [*Exercise Physiology for Fitness, Performance and Health.*]

Rosenberg, I. H. 2011. Sarcopenia: Origins and clinical relevance. *Clin Geriatr Med* 27:337-339.

Ruwer, S. L.; Rossi, A. G.; Simon, L. F. 2005. Equilíbrio no Idoso. *Rev. Bras. Otorrinolaringol.* 71 (3). [Balance in the Elderly]

Safons, M. P.; Balsamo, S. São Paulo: 2005. 2005. *Treinamento de força e envelhecimento*. São Paulo. [*Strength training and aging*]

Santos, L.; Ribeiro, A. S.; Schoenfeld, B. J.; Nascimento, M. A.; Tomeleri, C. M.; Souza, M. F.; et al. 2017. The improvement in walking speed induced by resistance training is associated with increased muscular strength but not skeletal muscle mass in older women. *European Journal of Sport Science*.

Seals, D. R.; Taylor, J. A.; Esler, M. D. 1994. Exercise and aging: autonomic control of the circulation. *Med. Sci. Sports Exerc.* 26:568-576.

Services., US Department of Health and Human. 2008. *Physical Activity Guidelines for Americans*.

Shepard, R. J. 2003. *Envelhecimento, Atividade Física e Saúde*. Edited by editora phorte. São Paulo. [*Aging, Physical Activity and Health*]

Shumway-Cook A.; Woollacott, M. H. 2007. *Motor Control: Translating Research into Clinical Practice*. Philadelphia: Lippincott Williams & Wilkins.

Silva, N. L.; Oliveira, R. B.; Fleck, S. J.; Leon, A. C. M. P.; Farinatti, P. 2014. Influence of strength training variables on strength gains in adults over 55 years-old: A meta-analysis of dose-response relationships. *Journal of Science and Medicine in Sport* 17:337-344.

Spirduso, W. W. 2005. *Dimensões físicas do envelhecimento*. São Paulo: Manole. [*Physical dimensions of aging*]

Tonet, A. C.; Nóbrega, O. T. 2008. Imunossenescência: a relação entre leucócitos, citocinas e doenças crônicas. *Rev. Bras. Geriatr. Gerotol.* 11 (2):259-273. [Immunosensescence: the relationship between leukocytes, cytokines and chronic diseases]

Toss, F.; Wiklund, P.; Nordström, P.; Nordström, A. (2012. Body composition and mortality risk in later life. *Age and Ageing* 41 (5):677-681.

BIOGRAPHICAL SKETCH

Eduardo Borba Neves

Affiliation: Brazilian Army Sports Commission (CDE, Rio de Janeiro, Brazil) and Universidade Tecnológica Federal do Paraná (UTFPR, Curitiba, Brazil)

Education: PhD in Biomedical Engineering

Research and Professional Experience: Eduardo Borba Neves is Colonel of the Brazilian Army, PhD in Biomedical Engineering and PhD in Public Health. He is with the Brazilian Army Sports Commission and with Graduate Program in Biomedical Engineering at the Federal Technological University of Paraná. His major research interests are in the fields of health diagnostic, physical fitness, thermal imaging and therapeutic technologies.

Publications from the Last 3 Years:

Articles in Scientific Journals

1) Fortes García, Rafael Chieza; Melo De Oliveira, Rafael; Martínez, Eduardo Camilo; Borba Neves, Eduardo. VO2 Estimation Equation Accuracy to Young Adults. *Archivos de Medicina* (Manizales), v. 20, p. 33-39, 2020.

2) Lima E Silva, L.; Neves, E.; Silva, J.; Alonso, L.; Vale, R.; Nunes, R. The haemodynamic demand and the attributes related to the displacement of the soccer referees in the moments of decision/intervention during the matches. *International Journal of Performance Analysis in Sport,* v. 20, p. 1-12, 2020.
3) Silva, Flávia Da; Yamaguchi, Bruna; Almeida, Karielly Cássia De; Costin, Ana Claudia Martins Szczypior; Maltauro, Luciana; Neves, Eduardo Borba; Mélo, Tainá Ribas. Efeito Imediato, Agudo E Crônico Da Kinesio Taping® Associada À Terapia Neuromotora Intensiva Na Postura Sentada De Crianças Com Paralisia Cerebral. *Arquivos de Ciências Da Saúde Da UNIPAR,* V. 24, P. 47-52, 2020.
4) Soster Iede Shiguihara, Dryelle; Brandão Oselame, Gleidson; Borba Neves, Eduardo. Tecnologias para o Diagnóstico da Radiodermite: uma Revisão Sistemática. *Archivos de Medicina* (Manizales), v. 20, p. 1-18, 2020. [Technologies for the Diagnosis of Radiodermatitis: A Systematic Review]
5) Bernardo, Luciana Dias; Scheeren, Eduardo Mendonça; Marson, Runer Augusto; Neves, Eduardo Borba. Stabilometric changes due to exposure to firearm noise in the Brazilian Army. *Bioscience Journal,* v. 36, p. 1410-1421, 2020.
6) Pucci, G. C. M. F.; Neves, E. B.; Saavedra, F. J. F. Effect of Pilates Method on Physical Fitness Related to Health in the Elderly: A Systematic Review. *Revista Brasileira De Medicina Do Esporte* (Online), v. 25, p. 76-87, 2019.
7) Fortes, Marcos De Sá Rego; Rosa, Samir Ezequiel Da; Coutinho, Walmir; Neves, Eduardo Borba. Epidemiological study of metabolic syndrome in Brazilian soldiers. *Archives of Endocrinology Metabolism*, v. 63, p. In Press, 2019.
8) Menegassi, D. A.; Sabbag, Alexandre De Aguiar; Costa, A. R. C.; Maltauro, L.; Mélo, Tainá Ribas; Neves, Eduardo Borba. Terapia neuromotora intensiva melhora a composição corporal na paralisia cerebral e amiotrofia. *Revista Brasileira De Obesidade, Nutrição E Emagrecimento,* v. 13, p. 275-283, 2019. [Intensive neuromotor therapy improves body composition in cerebral palsy and

amyotrophy. *Brazilian Journal Of Obesity, Nutrition And Weight Loss*]

9) Lima E Silva, L.; Godoy, E. S.; Neves, E. B.; Vale, R. G. S.; Lopez, J. A. H.; Nunes, R. A. M. Heart rate and the distance performed by the soccer referees during matches: a systematic review. *Archivos De Medicina Del Deporte*, v. 36, p. 36-42, 2019.

10) Reis, Victor M.; Neves, Eduardo B.; Garrido, Nuno; Sousa, Ana; Carneiro, André L.; Baldari, Carlo; Barbosa, Tiago. Oxygen Uptake On-Kinetics during Low-Intensity Resistance Exercise: Effect of Exercise Mode and Load. *International Journal of Environmental Research and Public Health*, v. 16, p. 2524, 2019.

11) Magas, Viviane; Abreu De Souza, Mauren; Borba Neves, Eduardo; Nohama, Percy. Evaluation of thermal imaging for the diagnosis of repetitive strain injuries of the wrist and hand joints. *Research on Biomedical Engineering*, v. 35, p. 57-64, 2019.

12) Monteiro, E. R.; Vingren, J.; Correa Neto, V. G.; Neves, E B; Steele, J.; Novaes, J. S. Effects of Different between Test Rest Intervals in Reproducibility of the 10-Repetition Maximum Load Test: A Pilot Study with Recreationally Resistance Trained Men. *International Journal of Exercise Science*, v. 12, p. 932-940, 2019.

13) Farias, Edvaldo De; Neves, Eduardo Borba; Quaresma, Luis Felgueiras; Vilaça-Alves, José Manuel. Avaliação da qualidade de serviços em Centros de Fitness no Rio de Janeiro: proposta de instrumento específico para instrutores. *Podium: Sport, Leisure And Tourism Review*, v. 8, p. 151-173, 2019. [Evaluation of service quality in Fitness Centers in Rio de Janeiro: proposal for a specific instrument for instructors.]

14) Mélo, Tainá Ribas; Freitas, Jheniffer; Sabbag, Alexandre De Aguiar; Chiarello, Claudiana Renata; Neves, Eduardo Borba; Israel, Vera Lucia. Intensive Neuromotor Therapy improves motor skills of children with Cornelia de Lange Syndrome: case report. *Fisioterapia Em Movimento*, v. 32, p. e003244, 2019.

15) Leal, S. O.; Neves, E. B.; Mello, D. B.; Filgueiras, M. Q.; Dantas, E. M. Pain perception and thermographic analysis in patients with

chronic lower back pain submitted to osteopathic treatment. *Motricidade* (Santa Maria Da Feira), v. 15, p. 12-20, 2019.
16) Neves, E. B. Thermal Imaging in Sports: Athlete's Thermal Passport. *Motricidade (Santa Maria Da Feira),* v. 15, p. 4-5, 2019.
17) Mélo, Tainá Ribas; Yamaguchi, Bruna; Chiarello, Claudiana Renata; Costin, Ana Cláudia Szczypior; Erthal, Vanessa; Israel, Vera Lúcia; Neves, Eduardo Borba. Intensive neuromotor therapy with suit improves motor gross function in cerebral palsy: a Brazilian study. *Motricidade (Santa Maria Da Feira),* v. 13, p. 54-61, 2018.
18) Matos, Filipe; Neves, Eduardo Borba; Rosa, Claudio; Reis, Victor Machado; Saavedra, Francisco; Silva, Severiano; Vilaça-Alves, José. Effect of Cold Water Immersion on Elbow Flexors Muscle Thickness after Resistance Training. *Journal of Strength and Conditioning Research,* v. 32, p. 1-763, 2018.
19) Salamunes, Ana Carla Chierighini; Stadnik, Adriana Maria Wan; Neves, Eduardo Borba. Estimation of Female Body Fat Percentage Based on Body Circumferences. *Revista Brasileira De Medicina Do Esporte* (Online), v. 24, p. 97-101, 2018.
20) Santos, Norma Claudia De Macedo Souza; Neves, Eduardo Borba; Fortes, Marcos De Sá Rego; Martinez, Eduardo Camillo; Júnior, Orlando Da Costa Ferreira. The influence of combat simulation exercises on indirect markers of muscle damage in soldiers of the Brazilian army. *Bioscience Journal,* v. 34, p. 1051-1061, 2018.
21) Sabbag, Alexandre De Aguiar; Costin, Ana Claudia Martins Szczypior; Menegassi, Daniel Alves; Silva, Juliana Bertolino; Braga, Marina Marcondes; Neves, Eduardo Borba. Etapa puberal en niños con parálisis cerebral. *Revista Científica General José María Córdova,* v. 16, p. 81-91, 2018. [Pubertal stage in children with cerebral palsy. *General Scientific Journal José María Córdova*]
22) Goncalves, M. M.; Marson, R. A.; Fortes, M. S. R.; Neves, E. B; Rodrigues Neto, G.; Novaes, J. S. The relationship between handgrip strength and total muscle strength in the Brazilian army military personnel. *Medicina Dello Sport,* v. 71, p. 461-473, 2018.

23) Krueger, E.; Scheeren, E. M.; Rinaldin, C. D. P.; Lazzaretti, A. E.; Neves, E. B.; Nogueira Neto, G. N.; Nohama, P. Impact of Skinfold Thickness on Wavelet-Based Mechanomyographic Signal. *Facta Universitatis*, V. 16, p. 359-368, 2018.
24) Oliveira, M. C. N.; Melo, T. R.; Pol, Stéphani; Costin, Ana Claudia Martins Szczypior; Oliveira, F. C. N.; Neves, E. B. Terapia neuromotora intensiva promove ganhos de habilidades motoras grossas e manutenção da composição corporal em crianças com paralisia cerebral. *Revista Brasileira De Obesidade, Nutrição E Emagrecimento*, v. 12, p. 598-606, 2018. [Intensive neuromotor therapy promotes gains in gross motor skills and maintenance of body composition in children with cerebral palsy. *Brazilian Journal Of Obesity, Nutrition And Weight Loss*]
25) Uchôa, Paulo; Matos, Filipe; Neves, Eduardo Borba; Saavedra, Francisco; Rosa, Claudio; Reis, Victor Machado; Vilaça-Alves, José. Evaluation of two different resistance training volumes on the skin surface temperature of the elbow flexors assessed by thermography. *Infrared Physics & Technology*, v. 93, p. 178-183, 2018.
26) Neves, E. B.; Garcia, Rafael Chieza Fortes; De Oliveira, Rafael Melo; Martinez, Eduardo Camillo. Incidence rate of musculoskeletal injuries in Brazilian army. *Bioscience Journal*, p. 1744-1750, 2018.
27) Santos, L. C.; Cherem, E. H.; Azeredo, F. P.; Neves, E. B.; Oliveira, D. R.; Novaes, G. S.; Silva, A. J.; Novaes, J. S. Effects of different strength training programs in young males maximal strength and anthropometrics. *Motricidade (Santa Maria Da Feira)*, v. 14, p. 301-309, 2018.
28) Welter, D. L.; Neves, E. B.; Saavedra, F. J. F. Profile of practitioners of supervised physical exercise in the Southern region of Brazil. *Bioscience Journal* (UFU), v. 33, p. 209-218, 2017.
29) Sumini, K. L.; Oselame, G. B.; Oselame, C. S.; Dutra, Denecir De Almeida; Neves, E. B. Alimentação, risco cardiovascular e nível de atividade física em adolescentes. *Revista Brasileira de Obesidade,*

Nutrição e Emagrecimento, v. 11, p. 23-30, 2017. [Diet, cardiovascular risk and physical activity level in adolescents. *Brazilian Journal of Obesity, Nutrition and Weight Loss*]

30) Salamunes, Ana Carla Chierighini; Stadnik, Adriana Maria Wan; Neves, Eduardo Borba. The effect of body fat percentage and body fat distribution on skin surface temperature with infrared thermography. *Journal of Thermal Biology*, v. 66, p. 1-9, 2017.

31) Garrett, Camylla Aparecida; Oselame, Gleidson Brandão; Neves, Eduardo Borba. O uso da episiotomia no Sistema Único de Saúde Brasileiro: a percepção das parturientes. *Revista Saúde e Pesquisa*, v. 9, p. 453-459, 2017. [The use of episiotomy in the Brazilian Unified Health System: the perception of parturients. *Health and Research Magazine*]

32) Oselame, Gleidson Brandão; Sanches, Ionildo José; Kuntze, Alana; Neves, Eduardo Borba. Software for automatic diagnostic prediction of skin clinical images based on ABCD rule. *Bioscience Journal*, v. 33, p. 1065-1078, 2017.

33) Crivellaro, Jackeline; Almeida, Renan Moritz Varnier Rodrigues De; Wenke, Rodney; Neves, Eduardo Borba. Perfil De Lesões Em Pilotos De Parapente No Brasil E Seus Fatores De Risco. *Revista Brasileira de Medicina do Esporte*, v. 23, p. 270-273, 2017. [Profile of Injuries in Paragliding Pilots in Brazil and Their Risk Factors. *Brazilian Journal of Sports Medicine*]

34) Goncalves, M. M.; Marson, R. A.; Fortes, M. S. R.; Neves, E. B.; Novaes, J. S. The relationship between total muscle strength and anthropometric indicators in Brazilian Army military. *Revista Brasileira De Obesidade, Nutrição E Emagrecimento, V.* 11, p. 330-337, 2017.

35) Melo De Oliveira, Rafael; Carreiro Lermen, Daniel; Augusto Marson, Runer; Borba Neves, Eduardo. La influencia del calentamiento activo, con o sin estiramiento estático, sobre la fuerza muscular en militares brasileños. *Revista Científica General José María Córdova*, v. 15, p. 157-166, 2017. [The influence of active warm-up, with or without static stretching, on muscular strength in

Brazilian military personnel. *General Scientific Journal José María Córdova*]

36) Santos, Michele Caroline Dos; Krueger, Eddy; Neves, Eduardo Borba. Electromyographic analysis of postural overload caused by bulletproof vests on public security professionals. *Research on Biomedical Engineering*, v. 33, p. 175-184, 2017.

37) De Souza, Rodrigo Poderoso; Cirilo De Sousa, Maria Do Socorro; Neves, Eduardo Borba; Rosa, Claudio; Cruz, Igor Raineh Durães; Targino Júnior, Adenilson; Macedo, José Onaldo Ribeiro; Reis, Victor Machado; Vilaça-Alves, José. Acute effect of a fight of Mixed Martial Arts (MMA) on the serum concentrations of testosterone, cortisol, creatine kinase, lactate, and glucose. *Motricidade (Santa Maria Da Feira)*, v. 13, p. 30-37, 2017.

38) Ulbrich, G. D. S.; Oselame, Gleidson Brandão; Oliveira, E. M.; Neves, E. B. Motivadores da ideação suicida e a autoagressão em adolescentes. *Adolescência & Saúde*, v. 14, p. 40-46, 2017.

39) Neves, Eduardo Borba; Salamunes, Ana Carla Chierighini; De Oliveira, Rafael Melo; Stadnik, Adriana Maria Wan. Effect of body fat and gender on body temperature distribution. *Journal of Thermal Biology*, v. 70, p. 1-8, 2017.

40) Neves, Eduardo Borba; Eraso, Natalia Morales; Narváez, Yesenia Seña; Rairan, Fabian Steven Garay; Garcia, Rafael Chieza Fortes. Musculoskeletal Injuries in sergeants training courses from Brazil and Colombia. *Journal of Science and Medicine in Sport*, v. 20, p. S117, 2017.

41) Neves, Eduardo Borba. Physical fitness tests in Latin American Armies. *Journal of Science and Medicine in Sport*, v. 20, p. S60, 2017.

42) Neves, Eduardo Borba; Da Rosa, Samir Ezequiel; Fortes, Marcos De Sá Rego. Prevalence and anthropometric predictors of metabolic syndrome in the Brazilian military. *Journal of Science and Medicine in Sport*, v. 20, p. S158, 2017.

43) Neves, Eduardo Borba; Rouboa, Abel; Machado, Leandro. Technologies for Assessment of Training Effects on Health and

Performance. *The Open Sports Sciences Journal,* v. 10, p. 222-222, 2017.

44) Capitani, Gabriel; Sehnem, Eduardo; Rosa, Claudio; Matos, Filipe; Reis, Victor M.; Neves, Eduardo B. Osgood-schlatter Disease Diagnosis by Algometry and Infrared Thermography. *The Open Sports Sciences Journal,* v. 10, p. 223-228, 2017.

45) Oselame, Cristiane Da Silva; Oselame, Gleidson Brandão; De Matos, Oslei; Neves, Eduardo Borba. Equation to Fat Percentage Estimation in Women with Reduced Bone Mineral Density. *The Open Sports Sciences Journal*, v. 10, p. 251-256, 2017.

46) Zaar, Andrigo; Neves, Eduardo Borba; Rouboa, Abel Ilah; Reis, Victor Machado. Determinative Factors in the Injury Incidence on Runners: Synthesis of Evidence -Injuries on Runners-. *The Open Sports Sciences Journal,* v. 10, p. 294-304, 2017.

47) Neves, Eduardo Borba. Correlations between the simulated military tasks performance and physical fitness tests at high altitude. *Motricidade (Santa Maria Da Feira),* v. 13, p. 12-17, 2017.

In: Physical Fitness and Exercise
Editor: Quinzia Trevisano

ISBN: 978-1-53618-521-8
© 2020 Nova Science Publishers, Inc.

Chapter 3

EFFECTS OF HIGH-INTENSITY RESISTANCE TRAINING ON OXIDATIVE STRESS

Eduardo Borba Neves[1,*], Danielli Braga de Mello[2], Rogério Santos de Aguiar[3], Juliana Brandão Pinto de Castro[3] and Rodrigo Gomes de Souza Vale[3,4]

[1]BrazilianArmy Sports Commission, CDE, Rio de Janeiro, Brazil, and Universidade Tecnológica Federal do Paraná, UTFPR, Curitiba, Brazil
[2]Physical Education College of the Brazilian Army, EsEFEx, Rio de Janeiro, Brazil
[3]State University of Rio de Janeiro, PPGCEE, IEFD, UERJ, Brazil
[4]Estácio de Sá University, UNESA, Cabo Frio/RJ, Brazil

ABSTRACT

This chapter presents the effects of Oxidative Stress (OS) in skeletal muscle during high-intense resistance training (HIRT). To this end, the following topics will be discussed: high-intense resistance training,

---

[*] Corresponding Author's E-mail: neveseb@gmail.com.

Oxidative stress, effects of high-intensity resistance training in skeletal muscle, definition of oxidative stress and reactive oxygen species (ROS), antioxidant defense system, and some final considerations. HIRT results in oxidative damage to macromolecules in blood and skeletal muscle. During HIRT, the metabolic rate in active skeletal muscle increases more than 100 times when compared to the levels at rest. The associated increase in oxygen consumption raises the ROS-s rate in skeletal muscle that have an impact on reducing muscle strength production. ROS produced during exercise leads to increased expression of endogenous antioxidants. These antioxidant molecules have the function of preventing the negative effects of ROS on the muscles, neutralizing free radicals. Also, ROS seems to be involved in the adaptation induced by the exercise of the muscle phenotype.

Keywords: resistance training, oxidative stress, exercise, biochemistry

HIGH-INTENSITY RESISTANCE TRAINING

According to American College of Sports Medicine (2018) the physical fitness is composed of various elements that can be grouped into health-related and skill-related components and the muscle strength (the ability of muscle to exert force) and resistance (the ability of muscle to continue to perform without fatigue) is one of them. Traditionally, each muscle group should be trained for a total of two to four sets. The sets maybe derived from the same exercise or from a combination of exercises affecting the same muscle group. The resistance training intensity and number of repetitions performed with each set are inversely related. That is, the greater the intensity or resistance, the fewer the number of repetitions that will need to be completed. To improve muscular strength to complete 8–12 repetitions should be performed.

Muscular strength development is underpinned by a combination of several morphological and neural factors. The usually strength methods that may be used to develop the strength-power characteristics are: bodyweight exercise, machine-based exercise, plyometrics, weightlifting derivatives, eccentric training, potentiation complexes, unilateral exercise, bilateral exercise, variable resistance, kettlebell training, ballistic training (Suchomal et al. 2018).

The resistance training (RT) has some synonyms in the literature, such as: strength training, endurance training or muscle strength training. And it consists of strength exercises which involve overcoming a resistance load (Bompa 2001).

The RT can have different levels of intensity. In this sense, the intensity refers to the level or degree of effort to which the individual is submitted during a determined training period or a training session. The increasing in the intensity of training requires a higher demand on organic systems, including the endocrine and muscular system (Weineck 2003).

The High Intensity Interval Training (HIIT) is also used for muscular strength and hypertrophy. The HIIT is usually defined as exercise consisting of repeated bouts of high-intensity work performed above the lactate threshold or critical speed/power, interspersed by periods of low-intensity exercise or complete rest (Laursen 2020).

Skeletal muscle is a highly specialized tissue that has excellent plasticity in response to stimuli, such as physical exercise and training (Steinbacher and Eckl 2015). Repetitive muscle contractions performed during high-intense resistance training (HIRT) raise the metabolic rate by active skeletal muscle more than 100 times the resting level that produces a variety of phenotypic and physiological responses (Azizbeigi et al. 2015).

These responses to prolonged or intense muscle contractile activity alter the physiological aspects of muscle fibers that predispose these fibers to higher rates of oxidative stress (OS) (Ferreira e Reid 2008). Thus, increasing oxygen consumption in muscle fibers decreases intracellular oxygen levels during exercise, which can promote an increase in OS (Clanton 2007; Powers et al. 2011). In addition, an increase in muscle temperature can raise the pressure of carbon dioxide (CO_2) and reduce pH. These factors, related to exercise, can stimulate the production of reactive oxygen species (ROS) in the muscle (Arbogast and Reid 2004; Powers et al. 2011).

ROS are not only released in muscle, but also in endothelial and immune cells to stimulate new adaptations during RT (Azizbeigi et al. 2015). These adaptations include the synthesis of cytokines, such as tumor necrosis factor

- Alpha (TNF-α) and interleukin-6 (IL-6) (Kosmidou et al.2002) that are affected by the intensity of muscle contraction (Azizbeigi et al. 2015). On the other hand, about 30% of circulating IL-6 comes from adipose tissue (Mohamed-Ali, Pinkney and Coppack 1998). But among several systemic inflammation markers, TNF-α and IL-6 are the most frequently measured, regardless of the stimulus to produce cytokines circulating in the human body (Donges et al. 2010).

ROS extensions and sources differ based on the type of physical exercise practiced by the contraction of skeletal muscles (Steinbacher and Eckl 2015; He et al. 2016). Moderate levels of ROS are necessary to produce muscle strength. However, excess ROS can lead to muscle fatigue and contractile dysfunction (Powers, Nelson and Hudson 2011).

To prevent ROS negative effects, antioxidant agents are transported to the muscles to neutralize free radicals. Therefore, there is evidence that oxidative stress has positive and negative effects on the muscle skeletal cells contraction. The adverse effects, such as reduced strength generation and increased muscle atrophy, seem to occur particularly after strenuous, non-regular exercise. In contrast, regular training has positive effects, influencing cellular processes that lead to the increased antioxidants expression.

EFFECTS OF HIGH-INTENSITY RESISTANCE TRAINING IN SKELETAL MUSCLE

Physical activity demands an increase in energy production from the musculoskeletal system. Depending on the training stimulus, a greater contribution from one of the three energy systems occurs:

1) the *phosphocreatine–creatine* kinase *system*, which is another chemical component that has a high energy phosphate bond.
2) the glycogen-lactic acid system uses the glycogen stored in the muscle that can be broken down into glucose, which is then used as energy. The initial stage of this process, called glycolysis, occurs

without the use of oxygen and, therefore, is called anaerobic metabolism.
3) the aerobic system. During glycolysis, each glucose molecule is divided into two molecules of pyruvic acid and energy is released to form four molecules of ATP for each original glucose molecule (Guyton and Hall 2011).

These energy systems are the processes by which ATP is produced and available to the muscle performance during contraction (McArdle, Katch and Katch, 2008).

Dynamic muscle contractions performed during the HIRT are composed of two phases: the concentric and the eccentric. These muscle actions are most performed during general population training that mainly uses free weights and weight machines (Bloomer 2008). And the increased contractile activity of skeletal muscle during exercise leads to a variety of physiological and biochemical adaptations in muscle tissue, including mitochondrial biogenesis, angiogenesis, changes in active myofibrils and ROS production.

Concentric muscle actions require a higher energy cost compared to eccentric actions (Dudley et al. 1991). But eccentric actions are primarily responsible for muscle damage and can generate ROS through lipid peroxidation and DNA oxidation.

The HIRT can induce oxidation and stress state, by an increase in oxidized molecules in a variety of tissues and body fluids. The extent of oxidation is dependent on the exercise protocol, intensity, and duration, and is specifically related to the degree of oxidant production. For example, on HIRT, there is an increase in oxygen consumption in muscle fibers, which leads to a decrease in intracellular oxygen levels during exercise, and an increase in ROS production (Clanton 2007; Richardson et al. 1995).

McBride et al. (1998) demonstrated that an HIRT protocol increases the production of ROS by analyzing methylmalonic acid (MMA) in blood plasma after exercise. Bailey et al. (2004) and Hovman et al. (2007) also demonstrated that an HIRT protocol increases the production of ROS analyzing blood plasma methylmalonic acid (MMA) after exercise, as well as reported an increase in lipid peroxidation after an acute HIRT. But

McAnulty et al. (2005) and Bloomer et al. (2007) observed no change in lipid peroxidation after HIRT.

Bloomer et al. (2005) stated that carbonyl proteins levels are increased after HIRT and post 24 hours. These data indicate that the production of ROS can increase even more for several times hours after HIRT, possibly mediated by changes in calcium homeostasis, as well as an increase in neutrophil (Quindry et al. 2003), both contributing to the increase in the production of ROS and that can lead to muscle damage.

In addition to the oxidation of lipids and proteins, DNA oxidation was measured after HIRT in two investigations (Bloomer et al. 2005; Bloomer et al. 2007). In both studies, no change was observed in DNA oxidation measured by 8-hydroxydeoxyguanosine serum. It is possible that DNA is better protected against oxidative stress than lipids and proteins, or perhaps due to the ability of DNA to undergo rapid repair once oxidized (Bloomer 2008).

In addition to the previously described effects of exercise on antioxidant enzymes activities, resistance training leads to adaptations of the cardiovascular and muscular system. In this sense, Irrcher et al. (2002) and Yan et al. (2011) found important responses at the intramyocellular level that include increases in the size and number of mitochondria, as well as in enzyme activities that facilitates the fatty acids oxidation (van Loon et al. 2006).

Olesen, Kiilerich and Pilegaard (2010) and Kang e Ji (2013) demonstrated that the receptor activated by peroxisome-activated *gamma* coactivator *1-alpha* (PGC-1α) is a key regulator of changes induced by HIRT in slow muscle fibers, as well as in protection against muscle atrophy. Activation of PGC-1 is likely to occur by phosphorylation of the PGC-1 protein and by mitogen-activated protein kinases (MAPK) in conjunction with nuclear factor-kappa B (NF-κB) (Wright et al. 2007), both known as ROS (Dodd et al. 2010; Derbre et al. 2012).

The PGC-1αhas been shown to regulate the metabolism of lipids and carbohydrates and improve the capacity of muscle fibers by increasing the quantity and activity of mitochondria through the positive regulation of nuclear respiratory factors (NRF-1/2) and mitochondrial transcription factor

A (TFAM) (Koves et al. 2005). In addition, PGC-1α regulates the genes involved in muscle fiber type (Steinbacher and Eckl 2015).

Structural changes mediated by ROS in lipids, proteins and DNA can be important for membrane remodeling, protein renewal, gene expression or epigenetic regulation. Therefore, this indicates that ROS are generated continuously in the contraction of skeletal muscle, in the processes of sarcopenia and hypertrophy.

The HIRT may increase the activities of superoxide dismutase (SOD) and glutathione peroxidase (GPx) in exercised muscles and plasma (Azizbeigi et al. 2014). This magnitude of exercise-mediated changes in SOD or GPx activities depends on the intensity and duration of exercise and the high intensity exercise can lead to higher GPx muscle activity than low intensity one (Fisher et al. 2011).

Likewise, long duration exercises (60 min/day or more) increases muscle GPx function more than short sessions exercises (30 min/day) (He et al. 2016). The increase in SOD and GPx function induced by exercise is specific to the muscle fiber type. Usually, a greater increase in skeletal muscles is observed, mainly composed of highly oxidative fibers (Ferraro et al. 2014).

The micro muscular injuries induced by strenuous exercises affect the immune cells and lead to a rapid formation of ROS and subsequent oxidative damage (Steinbacher and Eckl 2015). Thus, untrained individuals are more prone to the damaging effects exerted by oxidative stress, while trained individuals typically experience diminished effects due to increased oxidative tolerance (He et al. 2016).

The repetitive movements of intense effort, as in HIRT, and lead to muscle injuries (Barbe and Barr 2006), which range from minor damage with minimal loss of muscle function to major damage, which can lead to more serious complications as disrupts the components of the cellular cytoskeleton or leads to damage to the sarcolemma, which leads to loss of plasma permeability (Torres, Appell and Duarte 2006).

In addition, HIRT promotes damage to intracellular components, which results in biochemical changes with high ROS production and consequently, in reduction of muscle fibers to contract and relax (Silva et al. 2011; Silva et al. 2014). On the other hand, damage to muscle fibers is accompanied by the recruitment of phagocytic cells, such as macrophages and, although this process is essential for tissue repair, it involves the release of substantial amounts of ROS (Thirupathi and Pinho 2018).

However, the effects of ROS on injured tissues depend on the tissue antioxidant capacity (Pinho et al. 2017). The increase in ROS production, without an efficient and concomitant antioxidant system, promotes oxidative damage in cellular biomolecules and muscle contractile dysfunction. In this sense, the degree of alteration or regulation of the antioxidant system can determine the effectiveness of muscle repair, as well as the redox balance in muscle tissue.

In addition, the oxidation of ryanodine receptors that form intracellular calcium channels, which promotes muscle contractures (Salama, Menshikova and Abramson 2000), can lead to oxidative damage derived from two parental molecules - superoxide and nitric oxide (Powers and Jackson, 2008). Superoxide anions are denatured in cells to form hydrogen peroxide, hydroxyl radical and other low molecular weight oxidants located in the ERO cascade (Asmus and Bonifacic 2000).

Likewise, mitochondrial enzymes needed for energy production (for example, succinate dehydrogenase, cytochrome oxidase) are susceptible to oxidation (Bloomer 2008; Haycock et al. 1996). The oxidative damage in triphosphate phosphate adenosine pumps can decrease uptake of calcium through the sarcoplasmic reticulum, leading to an imbalance in calcium homeostasis and reducing muscle contractility (Bloomer 2008; Scherer and Deamer 1986).

The aging can also accelerate the rate of contraction-induced ROS production. About 2% to 5% of the total oxygen consumed by mitochondria (often cited as the predominant source of ROS in muscle cells) impact an electron reduction with the generation of superoxide (Powers, Nelson, and Hudson 2011).

As the contractile activity is directly related to increased oxygen consumption by the increased of mitochondrial respiration (Muller, Liu and Van Remmen 2004), this implies a 50 to 100 times increase in skeletal muscle superoxide generation during HIRT (Urso and Clarkson 2003).

In this context, evidence indicates more ROS are produced by mitochondria basal state than to the active state when muscle contraction increases the mitochondrial ADP levels due to the rapid breakdown of ATP (Kavazis et al. 2009).

DEFINITION OF OXIDATIVE STRESS AND REACTIVE OXYGEN SPECIES (ROS)

The term "oxidative stress" was first defined as "a disturbance in the antioxidant system" (Gerschman et al. 1954). Although this definition has been widely accepted for years, this description of oxidative stress is criticized by some authors, who propose other meanings for this term (Davies et al. 1982; Hammeren et al. 1992; Sen and Packer 1996; Sies and Cadenas 1985).

The researchers observed the complexity of cell redox balance. Thus, the term "oxidative stress" defines a simple pro-oxidant *versus* the definition of an antioxidant. This way, the description of an "oxidizing stress" is useful only if the molecular details of the redox imbalance are known (Azzi, Davies e Kelly 2004; Jones 2006). To refine the meaning of oxidative stress, it was suggested that this term be redefined as "an interruption in redox signaling and control" (Jones 2006).

However, studies related to the production sites of ROS in the contraction of skeletal muscles have remained a controversial topic for more than three decades. During the 1980s and 1990s, it was widely assumed that mitochondria were the dominant site of ROS production in muscle contraction (Pearson et al. 2014; Sakellariou et al. 2014). In the past, it was difficult to discern sub-cellular sources of ROS in muscle contraction due to inadequate analytical techniques available to study this issue (Pearson et al. 2014).

Nevertheless, more recent studies indicate that, during HIRT, mitochondria are not the dominant source of ROS (Goncalves et al. 2015; Sakellariou et al. 2014) and that nicotinamide adenine dinucleotide phosphate oxidase (NADPH) oxidase (NOX), and xanthine oxidase (XO) appear to play a key role in the production of ROS induced by muscle contraction (Sakellariou et al. 2014). In fact, mitochondria produce more ROS at rest than adenosine diphosphate (ADP) stimulated by HIRT (Powers, Nelson, and Hudson 2011; Goncalves et al. 2015).

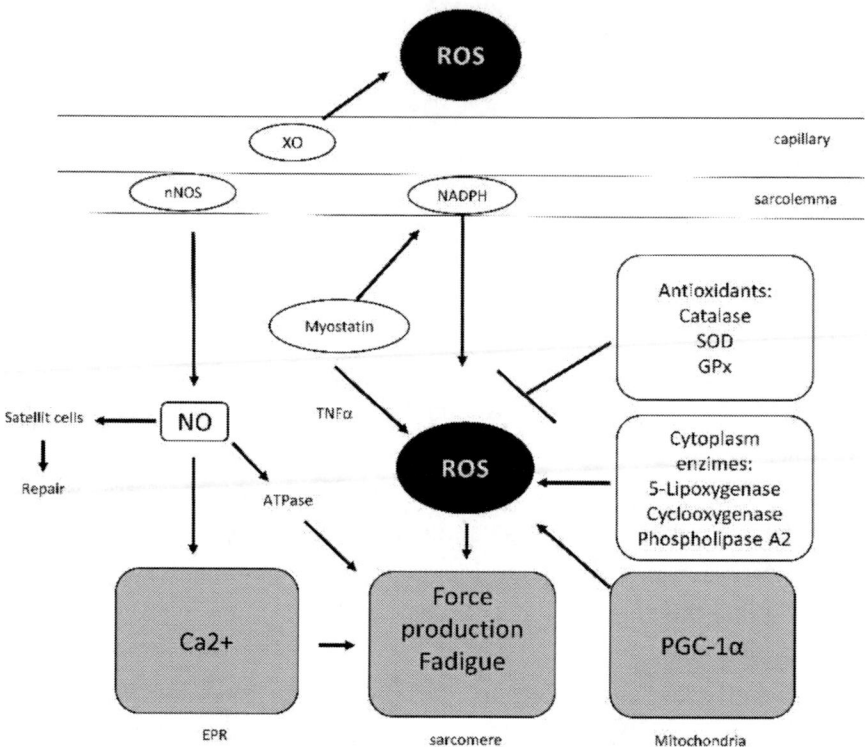

Figure 1. Potential sources of reactive oxygen species (ROS) in skeletal muscle.

Therefore, ROS are released as by-products of mitochondrial breathing, which is in the resting state and enters the active state when muscle contractions begin characterized by an increase in mitochondrial ADP levels due to the rapid breakdown of adenosine triphosphate (ATP). The rate of oxygen ($O_2\cdot^-$) production is generally higher in basal mitochondrial respiration than in the active state in skeletal muscle. In Figure 1, it is suggested that mitochondria may not be the main source of ROS for muscles during exercise (Powers and Jackson 2008; Kavazis et al. 2009; Sakellariou et al. 2013).

The main endogenous sources of ROS in skeletal muscle include mitochondria, NOX, XO, and lipoxygenases (Steinbacher and Eckl 2015). Under physiological conditions, ROS are released as by-products of cellular respiration through mitochondria. Consequently, mitochondrial derivatives ($O_2 \cdot -$) can be seen in both resting muscle and during exercise (Sakellariou et al. 2014).

The rate of O_2 production is normally higher in basal mitochondrial breathing than in the active state in skeletal muscle. Hence, it may be that mitochondria are not the main source of ROS in muscles during exercise (Kavazis et al. 2009; Powers and Jackson 2008; Sakellariou et al. 2014).

On the other hand, NOX is an important ROS generator during muscle contractions, contributing to a greater extent of cytosolic than mitochondria (Powers et al. 2011; Steinbacher and Eckl 2015). Additionally, NOX is a flavoprotein enzyme that is activated by calcium, free fatty acids, protein-protein interactions, and post-translational modifications. NOX uses NADPH as electron donors (Brandes et al. 2014). It is these transmembrane proteins in the transverse tubules and sarcoplasmic reticulum that carry out electron transport across biological membranes to reduce oxygen to superoxide or H_2O_2 (Brandes et al. 2014).

Shkryl et al. (2009) understood that members of the NOX family contribute to the production of cytosolic superoxide in skeletal muscle both at rest and during contractile activity to a greater extent than mitochondria. NOX generated by ROS activates ryanodine receptors (RyR), which leads to an intracellular release of Ca^{2+} (Hidalgo et al. 2006).

Diversely, Espinosa et al. (2009) found that insulin induces ROS generation through NOX activation and that ROS is important for intracellular Ca^{2+} increase mediated by inositol triphosphate receptors (InsP3R).

During intense exercise in which large amounts of ATP are consumed, hypoxanthine and xanthine levels are rising and serve as substrates for XO to generate ROS (Radak et al. 2013). XO is a cytosolic molybdoflavoenzyme, which is recognized as a key enzyme in purine catabolism. Purine catalyzes the hydroxylation of hypoxanthine to xanthine and xanthine uric acid (Harrison 2002).

In muscle, XO is present in the cytosol and also in the associated endothelial cells (Powers e Jackson, 2008). After muscle contraction, XO activity is significantly increased and leads to an increase in lipid peroxidation, oxidation, muscle damage, and edema (Judge and Doldd 2013).

Other factors, such as phospholipase A2 (PLA2) enzymes, have demonstrated the stimulation of NOX to produce ROS. PLA2 also facilitates the renewal of phospholipids and releases arachidonic acid (a substrate for lipoxygenases), leading to the further formation of ROS and damage related to lipid peroxidation (Steinbacher and Eckl 2015).

These ROS molecules are highly reactive and can cause deleterious effects in the body, such as the activation of mitochondrial biogenesis, fiber type transformation, and angiogenesis. Together, these effects tend to reduce the ability to generate muscle strength (Steinbacher and Eckl 2015).

In this sense, untrained individuals are more prone to the harmful effects exerted by enhanced oxidative stress, while trained individuals typically experience diminished effects due to increased oxidative tolerance (Steinbacher and Eckl, 2015).

Aging or muscle pathophysiological states are also associated with elevated ROS and contractile dysfunction (Steinbacher and Eckl, 2015). For instance, Palomero et al. (2013) and Vasilaki and Jackson (2013) observed a higher generation of endogenous oxidants in skeletal muscle fiber isolated from old mice compared to young mice at rest. It is suggested that such changes in ROS levels can be attributed to chronic muscle inactivity, which provides a possible explanation for the overproduction of ROS related to age in the muscle (Talbert et al. 2013; Vasilaki and Jackson 2013).

Moreover, in disease states, such as muscular dystrophy, simple contractions of stretching can lead to significant muscle damage associated with ROS generation, through increased activation of NOX and cytosolic Ca^{2+} levels (Whitehead et al. 2010).

In view of the exposed evidence, ROS are generated continuously at rest in muscle contraction and are necessary for the physiological function to occur in skeletal muscle. In addition to the production of mitochondrial ROS, XO and NADPH, stimulated by HIRT, are the main sources of ROS.

ANTIOXIDANT DEFENSE SYSTEM

The role of antioxidants is to slow or stop these chain reactions by removing free radicals or inhibiting other oxidation reactions. Thus, antioxidants are often reducing agents, such as polyphenols or thiols (Duarte and Lunec 2005).

Muscle activity leads to a strong increase in ROS production. Simultaneously, the body's antioxidant defense mechanisms are activated. To maintain adequate cell signaling, several radical-destroying enzymes are likely to maintain a limited level of ROS within the cell (Adwas et al. 2019). However, when the ROS level exceeds this limit, it can lead to irreversible damage to essential macromolecules, DNA, proteins, and lipids, initiating carcinogenesis (Imlay 2003).

Therefore, ROS concentrations must be controlled by several defense mechanisms, which also involve several antioxidant enzymes, such as glutathione and detoxifying vitamins C and E. These antioxidant molecules can neutralize free radicals, accepting the unpaired electron. Hence, they inhibit the oxidation of other molecules (Steinbacher and Eckl 2015).

Depending on the rate of oxygen consumption, cells express different levels of antioxidant enzymes, including mitochondrial antioxidant manganese superoxide dismutase (MnSOD, SOD2), cytosolic copper-zinc superoxide dismutase (Cu, Zn-SOD, SOD1), glutathione peroxidase (GPx), catalase (CAT), and non-enzymatic antioxidant glutathione (GSH)(Ji 1999).

Catalase is another important antioxidant enzyme. Nevertheless, it remains controversial whether chronic physical exercise can affect the expression or activity of this enzyme, as previous studies have reported mixed results (Brooks et al. 2008; Liberali, Wilhelm Filho, and Petroski 2016; Vincent et al. 2000). These results proposed several important ways of mediating adaptive responses to physical training (Csala et al. 2015; Morris et al. 2008; Samjoo et al. 2013). Therefore, they suggest that the mitochondrial ROS generated during intense regular exercise is necessary for the activation of the primary signaling pathways associated with muscle adaptation, such as antioxidants (Yavari et al. 2015).

Among the antioxidants, the nuclear factor erythroid 2-related factor 2(Nrf2) is a transcription factor with redox detection. In this sense, Nrf2 is the main antioxidant regulator among other cytoprotective cofactors responsible for the improved antioxidant defense system (Muthusamy et al. 2012). Regulated Nrf2 expression occurs after high-intensity exercise (Gounder et al. 2012).

The antioxidant defense mechanisms (non-enzymatic and enzymatic) with the function: 1) Blocking the production of free radicals; 2) Elimination of oxidants; 3) Conversion of toxic free radicals into less toxic substances; 4) Blocking the production of secondary substances, toxic metabolites, and inflammation mediators; 5) Blocking the chain propagation of secondary oxidants; 6) Repair of wound molecules; 7) Initiation and increase of the endogenous antioxidant defense system work together to protect the body against ROS(Adwas et al. 2019).

Trapp, Knez, and Sinclair (2010) reported that the best-known antioxidants are vitamins, which can be obtained quickly through natural foods such as vegetables and fruits. Indeed, vegetarians have been shown to have higher levels of endogenous vitamin than omnivorous due to antioxidant-rich diets, providing effective protection against exercise-induced oxidative stress (Rauma andMykkänen 2000; Trapp,Knez, and Sinclair 2010). These foods are often used by athletes to improve performance and promote accelerated muscle recovery, as the intake of antioxidant vitamins demonstrates potential prophylactic effects (Margaritis and Rousseau 2008).

Accordingly, the development of a natural antioxidant diet associated with individualized exercises in different populations of active subjects and athletes could minimize the action of oxidative stress on the body induced by intense training.

CONCLUSION

Oxidative stress induced by exercise and the effects of ROS have been widely studied in recent decades. Despite the increasingly sophisticated research in the study of ROS in skeletal muscle, these are generated continuously in the contraction of skeletal muscle and their presence is mandatory for normal physiological function. HIRT promotes increased ROS production in skeletal muscle, which leads to the need to seek strategies for modulating these substances with antioxidants. In addition to the production of mitochondrial ROS, XO and NADPH are the main sources of ROS. Excessive ROS production, in addition to antioxidant defense capacity, after exhaustive exercise in trained or untrained individuals can adversely affect phenotypic and physiological adaptive responses.

REFERENCES

Adwas, A. A., A. S. I. Elsayed, A. E. D. AzabandF. A. Quwaydir. 2019. "Oxidative stress and antioxidant mechanisms in the human body." *Journal of Applied Biotechnology & Bioengineering* 6, no. 1 (fevereiro): 43-7.10.1097/WOX.0b013e3182439613.

Andrade, F. H., M. B. Reid, D. G. Allenand H. Westerblad. 1998. Effect of hydrogen peroxide and dithiothreitol on contractile function of single skeletal muscle fibres from the mouse. *Journal of Physiology* 509, no. 2 (junho): 565-75. https://doi.org/10.1111/j.1469-7793.1998.565bn.x.

Arbogast, S. and M. B. Reid. 2004. "Oxidant activity in skeletal muscle fibers is influenced by temperature, CO_2 level, and muscle-derived nitric oxide." *American Journal of Physiology-Regulatory, Integrative and Comparative Physiology* 287, no. 4 (outubro): 698-705. https://doi.org/10.1152/ajpregu.00072.2004.

Asmus, K. D. and M. Bonifacic. 2000. "Free radical chemistry." Em *Handbook of oxidants and antioxidants*, 3-54. Amsterdam: Elsevier.

Austin, S., E. Klimcakova and J. St-Pierre. 2011. "Impact of PGC-1α on the topology and rate of superoxide production by the mitochondrial electron transport chain." *Free Radical Biology and Medicine* 51, no. 12 (dezembro): 2243-8. https://doi.org/10.1016/j.freeradbiomed.2011.08.036.

Azizbeigi, K., M. A. Azarbayjani, S. Atashakcand S. R. Stannardd. 2015. "Effect of moderate and high resistance training intensity on indices of inflammatory and oxidative stress." *Research in Sports Medicine* 23, no. 1 (fevereiro): 73-87. https://doi.org/10.1080/15438627.2014.975807.

Azizbeigi, K., S. R. Stannard, S. Atashakand M. M. Haghighi. 2014. "Antioxidant enzymes and oxidative stress adaptation to exercise training: comparison of endurance, resistance, and concurrent training in untrained males." *Journal of Exercise Science & Fitness* 12, no. 1 (junho): 1-6. https://doi.org/10.1016/j.jesf.2013.12.001.

Azzi, A., K. J. A. Daviesand F. Kelly. 2004. "Free radical biology – terminology and critical thinking." *FEBS Letters* 558, no. 1–3 (janeiro): 3-6.https://doi.org/10.1016/S0014-5793(03)01526-6.

Bailey, D. M., I. S. Young, J. McEneny, L. Lawrenson, J. Kim, J. Bardenand R. S. Richardson. 2004. "Regulation of free radical outflow from an isolated muscle bed in exercising humans." *American Journal of Physiology-Heart and Circulatory Physiology* 287, no. 4 (outubro): 1689-99.https://doi.org/10.1152/ajpheart.00148.2004.

Barbe, M. F.andA. E. Barr. 2006. "Inflammation and the pathophysiology of work-related musculoskeletal disorders." *Brain, Behavior, and Immunity* 20, no. 5 (setembro): 423-9. https://doi.org/10.1016/j.bbi.2006.03.001.

Bloomer, R. J. 2008. "Effect of exercise on oxidative stress biomarkers." *Advances in Clinical Chemistry* 46: 1-50. https://doi.org/10.1016/s0065-2423(08)00401-0.

Bloomer, R. J., A. C. Fry, M. J. Falvoand C. A. Moore. 2007. "Protein carbonyls are acutely elevated following single set anaerobic exercise in resistance trained men." *Journal of Science and Medicine in Sport* 10, no. 6:411-7.

Bloomer, R. J., A. H. Goldfarb, L. Wideman, M. J. McKenzieand L. A. Consitt.2005. "Effects of acute aerobic and anaerobic exercise on blood markers of oxidative stress." *Journal of Strength & Conditioning Research* 19, no. 2 (maio): 276-85.

Bompa, T. O. 2001. *A periodização no treinamento esportivo*. São Paulo: Manole.

Brand, M. D. 2010. "The sites and topology of mitochondrial superoxide production." *Experimental Gerontology* 45, no. 7-8 (agosto): 466-72. https://doi.org/10.1016/j.exger.2010.01.003.

Brandes, R. P., N. Weissmann, K. Schröder. 2014. "Nox family NADPH oxidases: Molecular mechanisms of activation." *Free Radical Biology and Medicine* 76, 208-26. https://doi.org/10.1016/j.freeradbiomed.2014.07.046.

Brooks, S. V., A. Vasilaki, L. M. Larkin, A. McArdleand M. J. Jackson. 2008. "Repeated bouts of aerobic exercise lead to reductions in skeletal muscle free radical generation and nuclear factor kB activation." *Journal of Physiology* 586 (agosto): 3979-90. https://doi.org/10.1113/jphysiol.2008.155382.

Clanton, T. L. 2007. "Hypoxia-induced reactive oxygen species formation in skeletal muscle." *Journal of Applied Physiology* 102, no. 6 (junho):2379-88. https://doi.org/10.1152/japplphysiol.01298.2006.

Csala, M., T. Kardon, B. Legeza, B. Lizák, J. Mandl, E. Margittai et al. 2015. "On the role of 4-hydroxynonenalin health and disease." *Biochimica et Biophysica Acta (BBA) - Molecular Basis of Disease* 1852, no. 5, p. 826-38. https://doi.org/10.1016/j.bbadis.2015.01.015.

Davies, K. J., A. T. Quintanilha, G. A. Brooks and L. Packer. 1982. "Free radicals and tissue damage produced by exercise." *Biochemical and Biophysical Research Communications* 107, no. 4 (agosto): 1198-1205.https://doi.org/10.1016/S0006-291X(82)80124-1.

Derbre, F., B. Ferrando, M. C. Gomez-Cabrera, F. Sanchis-Gomar, V. E. Martinez-Bello, G. Olaso-Gonzalez, et al. 2012. "Inhibition of xanthine oxidase by allopurinol prevents skeletal muscle atrophy: Role of p38 MAPKinase and E3 ubiquitin ligases." *PLoS One* 7, no. 10 (outubro):e46668.https://doi.org/10.1371/journal.pone.0046668.

Dodd, S. L., B. J. Gagnon, S. M. Senf, B. A. Hain and A. R. Judge. 2010. "ROS-mediated activation of NF-κB and Foxo during muscle disuse." *Muscle Nerve* 41, no. 1 (janeiro): 110-3. https://doi.org/10.1002/mus. 21526.

Donges, C. E., R. Duffieldand E. J. Drinkwater.2010. "Effects of resistance or aerobic exercise training on interleukin-6, C-reactive protein, and body composition." *Medicine & Science in Sports & Exercise* 42, no. 2 (fevereiro): 304-13. https://doi.org/10.1249/MSS.0b013e3181b117ca.

Duarte, T. L.and J. Lunec. 2005. "Review: When is an antioxidant not an antioxidant? A review of novel actions and reactions of vitamin C." *Free Radical Research* 39, no. 7: 671-86. http://dx.doi.org/10.1080/ 10715760500104025.

Dudley, G. A., P. A.Tesch, R. T. Harris, C. L. Golden and P. Buchanan.1991. "Influence of eccentric actions on the metabolic cost of resistance exercise." *Aviation Space and Environmental Medicine* 62, no. 7 (julho): 678-82.

Espinosa, A., A. García, S. Härtel, C. Hidalgo and E. Jaimovich.2009. "NADPH oxidase and hydrogen peroxide mediate insulin-induced calcium increase in skeletal muscle cells." *Journal of Biological Chemistry* 284 (janeiro): 2568-75.https://doi.org/10.1074/jbc.M8042 49200.

Favero, T. G., A. C.Zable, J. J. Abramson.1995. "Hydrogen peroxide stimulates the Ca2+ release channel from skeletal muscle sarcoplasmic reticulum." *Journal of Biological Chemistry* 270, no. 43 (outubro): 25557-63. https://doi.org/10.1074/jbc.270.43.25557.

Ferraro, E., A. M. Giammarioli, S. Chiandotto, I. Spoletiniand G. Rosano. 2014. "Exercise-induced skeletal muscle remodeling and metabolic adaptation: redox signaling and role of autophagy." *Antioxidants & Redox Signaling* 21, no. 1 (julho): 154-76. https://doi.org/10. 1089/ars.2013.5773.

Ferreira, L. F.and M. B. Reid. 2008. "Muscle-derived ROS and thiol regulation in muscle fatigue." *Journal of Applied Physiology* 104, no. 3 (março):853-60. https://doi.org/10.1152/japplphysiol.00953.2007.

Fisher, G., D. D. Schwartz, J. Quindry, M. D. Barberio, E. B. Foster, K. W. Jonesand D. D. Pascoe. 2011. "Lymphocyte enzymatic antioxidant responses to oxidative stress following high-intensity interval exercise." *Journal of Applied Physiology* 110, no. 3 (março): 730-7. https://doi.org/10.1152/japplphysiol.00575.2010.

Gerschman, R., D. L. Gilbert, S. W. Nye, P. Dwyer, W. O. Fenn. 1954. "Oxygen poisoning and x-irradiation: a mechanism in common." *Science* 119, no. 3097 (maio): 623-6. https://doi.org/10.1126/science.119.3097.623.

Goldhaber, J. I. and M. S. Qayyum.2008. "Oxygen free radicals and excitation-contraction coupling." *Antioxidants & Redox Signaling* 2, no. 1 (março): 55-64. https://doi.org/10.1089/ars.2000.2.1-55.

Gomez-Cabrera, M. C., Domenech, E., Vina, J. Moderate exercise is an antioxidant: Upregulation of antioxidant genes by training. *Free Radic. Biol. Med.* 2008, 44, 126–131. https://doi: 10.1016/j.freeradbiomed.2007.02.001.

Goncalves, R. L. S., C. L. Quinlan,I. V. Perevoshchikova, M. Hey-Mogensen e M. D. Brand. 2015. "Sites of superoxide and hydrogen peroxide production by muscle mitochondria assessed ex vivo under conditions mimicking rest and exercise." *Journal of Biological Chemistry* 290, no.1 (janeiro): 209-27. https://doi.org/10.1074/jbc.M114.619072.

Gounder, S. S., S. Kannan, D. Devadoss, C. J. Miller, K. J. Whitehead, S. J. Odelberg et al. 2012. "Impaired transcriptional activity of Nrf2inage-related myocardial oxidative stress is reversible by moderate exercise training." *PLoS ONE* 7, no. 9:e45697. https://doi.org/10.1371/journal.pone.0045697.

Guyton, A. C.and Hall, J. E. *Tratado de fisiologia médica*. 2011. Elsevier. 1089-1092. [*Treatise on medical physiology*.]

Hammeren, J., S. Powers, J. Lawler, D. Criswell, D. Martin, D. Lowenthal and M. Pollock. 1992. "Exercise training-induced alterations in skeletal muscle oxidative and antioxidant enzyme activity in senescent rats." *International Journal of Sports Medicine* 13, no. 5: 412-6. https://doi.org/10.1055/s-2007-1021290.

Harrison, R. 2002. "Structure and function of xanthine oxidoreductase: Where are we now?" *Free Radical Biology and Medicine* 33, no. 6 (setembro): 774-97. https://doi.org/10.1016/S0891-5849(02)00956-5.

Haycock, J. W., P. Jones, J. B. Harrisand D. Mantle. 1996. "Differential susceptibility of human skeletal muscle proteins to free radical induced oxidative damage: A histochemical, immunocytochemical and electron microscopical study in vitro." *Acta Neuropathologica* 92, no. 4: 331-40.https://doi.org/10.1007/s004010050527.

He, F., J. Li, Z. Liu, C. C. Chuang, W. Yang and L. Zuo. 2016. "Redox mechanism of reactive oxygen species in exercise." *Frontiers in Physiology* 7: 486. https://doi.org/10.3389/fphys.2016.00486.

Hidalgo, C., G. Sánchez, G. Barrientos and P. Aracena-Parks. 2006. "A transverse tubule NADPH oxidase activity stimulates calcium release from isolated triads via ryanodine receptor type 1 S-glutathionylation." *Journal of Biological Chemistry* 281 (setembro): 26473-82. https://doi.org/10.1074/jbc.M600451200.

Hovman, J. R., J. Im, J. Kang, C. M. Maresh, W. J. Kraemer, D. French, S. et al. 2007. "Comparison of low- and high-intensity resistance exercise on lipid peroxidation: Role of muscle oxygenation." *Journal of Strength and Conditioning Research* 21, no. 1 (janeiro): 118-22. https://doi.org/10.1519/00124278-200702000-00022.

Imlay, J. A. 2003. "Pathways of oxidative damage." *Annual Review of Microbiology* 57 (outubro): 395-418. https://doi.org/10.1146/annurev.micro.57.030502.090938.

Irrcher, I., P. J. Adhihetty, T. Sheehan, A. M. Josephand D. A. Hood. 2003. "PPARgamma coactivator-1alpha expression during thyroid hormone- and contractile activity-induced mitochondrial adaptations." *American Journal of Physiology-Cell Physiology* 284, no. 6 (junho): 1669-77.https://doi.org/10.1152/ajpcell.00409.2002.

Jackson, M. J. 2011. "Control of reactive oxygen species production in contracting skeletal muscle." *Antioxidants & Redox Signaling* 15, no. 9: 2477-86.https://doi.org/10.1089/ars.2011.3976.

Ji, L. L.1999. "Antioxidants and oxidative stress in exercise." *Proceedings of the Society for Experimental Biology and Medicine* 222, no. 3

(dezembro): 283-92. https://doi.org/10.1046/j.1525-1373.1999.d01-145.x.

Jones, D. P. 2006. "Redefining oxidative stress." *Antioxidants & Redox Signaling* 8, no. 9-10 (setembro): 1865-79. https://doi.org/10.1089/ars.2006.8.1865.

Judge, A. R. and S. L. Dodd. 2004. "Xanthine oxidase and activated neutrophils cause oxidative damage to skeletal muscle after contractile claudication." *American Journal of Physiology-Heart and Circulatory Physiology* 286, no. 1 (janeiro): 252-6. https://doi.org/10.1152/ajpheart.00684.2003.

Kang, C. and L. L. Ji. 2013. "Role of PGC-1α in muscle function and aging." *Journal of Sport and Health Science* 2, no. 2 (junho): 81-6. https://doi.org/10.1016/j.jshs.2013.03.005.

Kavazis, A. N., E. E. Talbert, A. J. Smuder, M. B. Hudson, W. B. NelsonandS. K. Powers. 2009. "Mechanical ventilation induces diaphragmatic mitochondrial dysfunction and increased oxidant production." *Free Radical Biology and Medicine* 46, no. 6 (março): 842-50. https://doi.org/10.1016/j.freeradbiomed.2009.01.002.

Kosmidou, I., T. Vassilakopoulous, A. Xagorari, S. Zakynthinos, A. Papapetropoulos and C. Roussos. 2002. "Production of interleukin-6 by skeletal my o tubes. Role of reactive oxygen species." *American Journal of Respiratory Cell and Molecular Biology* 26, no. 5: 587-93. https://doi.org/10.1165/ajrcmb.26.5.4598.

Koves, T. R., P. Li, J. An, T. Akimoto, D. Slentz, O. Ilkayeva, et al. 2005. "Peroxisome proliferator-activated receptor-γ co-activator 1α-mediated metabolic remodeling of skeletal myocytes mimics exercise training and reverses lipid-induced mitochondrial inefficiency." *Journal of Biological Chemistry* 280 (setembro):33588-98. https://doi.org/10.1074/jbc.M507621200.

Liberali, R., D. Wilhelm Filho and E. L. Petroski, 2016. "Aerobic and anaerobic training sessions promote antioxidant changes in young male soccer players." *Medical Express* 3, no. 1, p. 1-7. https://doi.org/10.5935/MedicalExpress.2016.01.07.

Laursen, P. and Buchheit, M. (2019). *Science and Application of High-Intensity Interval Training.* Human Kinetics.

Malech, H. L. and J. I. Gallin.1987. "Current concepts: immunology. Neutrophils in human diseases." *New England Journal of Medicine* 317, no. 11 (setembro): 687-94. https://doi.org/10.1056/NEJM19870 9103171107.

Margaritis, I. and A. S. Rousseau. 2008. "Does physical exercise modify antioxidant requirements?" *Nutrition Research Reviews* 21, no. 1 (junho): 3-12. https://doi.org/10.1017/S0954422408018076.

McAnulty, S. R., L. S. McAnulty, D. C. Nieman, J. D. Morrow, L. A. Shooter, S. Holmes, C. Hewardand D. A. Henson. 2005. "Effect of alpha-tocopherol supplementation on plasma homocysteine and oxidative stress in highly trained athletes before and after exhaustive exercise." *Journal of Nutritional Biochemistry* 16, no. 9 (setembro): 530-7. https://doi.org/10.1016/j.jnutbio.2005.02.001.

McArdle, W. D., Katch, F. I., and Katch, V. L. 2008. *Fisiologia do Exercício.* Rio de Janeiro. Guanabara Koogan.

McBride, J. M., W. J. Kraemer, T. Triplett-McBrideand W. Sebastianelli. 1998. "Effect of resistance exercise on free radical production." *Medicine & Science in Sports & Exercise* 30, no. 1 (janeiro): 67-72.

Michaelson, L. P., Shi, G., Ward, C. W. and Rodney, G. G. 2010. Potencial redox mitocondrial durante a contração em fibras musculares intactas. *Nervo Muscular* 42, 522-529. doi: 10.1002 / mus.21724. [Mitochondrial redox potential during contraction in intact muscle fibers.]

Mohamed-Ali, V., J. H. Pinkneyand S. W. Coppack. 1998. "Adipose tissue as an endocrine and paracrine organ." *International Journal of Obesity.* 22: 1145-58. https://doi.org/10.1038/sj.ijo.0800770.

Morris, R. T., M. J. Laye, S. J. Lees, R. S. Rector, J. P. Thyfaultand F. W. Booth. 2008. "Exercise induced attenuation of obesity, hyperinsulinemia, and skeletal muscle lipid peroxidation in the OLETF rat." *Journal of Applied Physiology* 104, no. 3 (março): 708-15. https://doi.org/10.1152/japplphysiol.01034.2007.

Muller, F. L., Y. Liu and H. Van Remmen. 2004. "Complex III releases superoxide to both sides of the inner mitochondrial membrane." *Journal of Biological Chemistry* 279, no. 47 (novembro): 49064-73. https://doi.org/10.1074/jbc.M407715200.

Muthusamy, V. R., S. Kannan, K. Sadhaasivam, S. S. Gounder, C. J. Davidson, C. Boeheme et al. 2012. "Acute exercise stress activates Nrf2/ARE signaling and promotes antioxidant mechanisms in the myocardium." *Free Radical Biology and Medicine* 52, no. 2 (janeiro): 366-76. https://doi.org/10.1016/j.freeradbiomed.2011.10.440.

Nemes, R., E. Koltai, A. W. Taylor, K. Suzuki, F. Gyoriand Z. Radak. 2018. "Reactive oxygen and nitrogen species regulate key metabolic, anabolic, and catabolic pathways in skeletal muscle." *Antioxidants* 7, no. 7 (julho): 85. https://doi.org/10.3390/antiox7070085.

Olesen, J., K. Kiilerichand H. Pilegaard, H. 2010. "PGC-1alpha-mediated adaptations in skeletal muscle." *Pflügers Archiv: European Journal of Physiology* 460, no. 1 (junho): 153-62. https://doi.org/10.1007/s00424-010-0834-0.

Palomero, J., Vasilaki, A., Pye, D., McArdle, A. and Jackson, M. J. (2013). O envelhecimento aumenta a oxidação da dicloridrofluoresceína em fibras musculares esqueléticas isoladas em repouso, mas não durante as contrações. *Sou. J. Physiol. Regul. Integr. Comp. Physiol.* 305, R351 – R358. doi: 10.1152 / ajpregu.00530.2012. [Aging increases the oxidation of dichlorohydrofluorescein in isolated skeletal muscle fibers at rest, but not during contractions.]

Pearson, T., T. Kabayo, R. Ng, J. Chamberlain, A. McArdleand M. J. Jackson. 2014. Skeletal muscle contractions induce acute changes in cytosolic superoxide, but slower responses in mitochondrial superoxide and cellular hydrogen peroxide. *PLoS One* 9, no. 5: e96378. https://doi.org/10.1371/journal.pone.0096378.

Pinho, R. A., D. M. Sepa-Kishi, G. Bikopoulos, M. V. Wu, A. Uthayakumar, A. Mohasses et al. 2017. "High-fat diet induces skeletal muscle oxidative stress in a fiber type-dependent manner in rats." *Free Radical Biology and Medicine* 110 (setembro): 381-9.https://doi.org/10.1016/j.freeradbiomed.2017.07.005.

Powers, S. K.and M. J. Jackson.2008. "Exercise-induced oxidative stress: Cellular mechanisms and impact on muscle force production."

Physiological Reviews 88, no. 4 (outubro): 1243-76. https://doi.org/10.1152/physrev.00031.2007.

Powers, S. K., L. L. Ji, A. N. Kavazisand M. J. Jackson. 2011. "Reactive oxygen species: impact on skeletal muscle." *Comprehensive Physiology* 1, no. 2 (abril): 941-69. https://doi.org/10.1002/cphy.c100054.

Powers, S. K., W. B. Nelsonand M. B. Hudson. 2011. "Exercise-induced oxidative stress in humans: Cause and consequences." *Free Radical Biology and Medicine* 51, no. 5 (setembro): 942-50.https://doi.org/10.1016/j.freeradbiomed.2010.12.009.

Quindry, J. C., W. L. Stone, J. King and C. E. Broeder. 2003. "The effects of acute exercise on neutrophils and plasma oxidative stress." *Medicine & Science in Sports & Exercise* 35, no. 7 (julho): 1139-45. https://doi.org/10.1249/01.MSS.0000074568.82597.0B.

Radak, Z., Z. Zhao, E. Koltai, H. Ohno and M. Atalay. 2013. "Oxygen consumption and usage during physical exercise: The balance between oxidative stress and ROS-dependent adaptive signaling." *Antioxidants & Redox Signaling* 18, no. 10 (abril): 1208-46. https://doi.org/10.1089/ars.2011.4498.

Rauma, A. L. and H. Mykkänen. 2000. "Antioxidant status in vegetarians versus omnivores." *Nutrition* 16, no. 2 (fevereiro): 111-9. https://doi.org/10.1016/s0899-9007(99)00267-1.

Richardson, R. S., E. A. Noyszewski, K. F. Kendrick, J. S. Leigh, P. D. Wagner. 1995. "Myoglobin O_2 desaturation during exercise. Evidence of limited O_2 transport." *Journal of Clinical Investigation* 96, no. 4 (outubro): 1916-26. https://doi.org/10.1172/JCI118237.

Sakellariou, G. K., A. Vasilaki, J. Palomero, A. Kayani, L. Zibrik, A. McArdle and M. J. Jackson. 2013. "Studies of mitochondrial and nonmitochondrial sources implicate nicotinamide adenine dinucleotide phosphate oxidase(s) in the increased skeletal muscle superoxide generation that occurs during contractile activity." *Antioxid Redox Signal* 18, no. 6 (fevereiro): 603-21. https://doi.org/10.1089/ars.2012.4623.

Salama, G., E. V. Menshikova and J. J. Abramson. 2000. "Molecular interaction between nitric oxide and ryanodine receptors of skeletal and cardiac sarcoplasmic reticulum." *Antioxidants & Redox Signaling* 2, no.1 (março): 5-16.https://doi.org/10.1089/ars.2000.2.1-5.

Samjoo, I. A., A. Safdar, M. J. Hamadeh, S. Rahaand M. A. Tarnopolsky. 2013. "The effect of endurance exercise on both skeletal muscle and systemic oxidative stress in previously sedentary obese men." *Nutrition & Diabetes* 3, no. 9 (setembro): e88. https://doi.org/10.1038/nutd.2013.30.

Scherer, N. M. And D. W. Deamer. 1986. "Oxidative stress impairs the function of sarcoplasmic reticulum by oxidation of sulfhydryl groups in the Ca^{2+}-ATPase." *Archives of Biochemistry and Biophysics* 246, no. 2 (maio): 589-601. https://doi.org/10.1016/0003-9861(86)90314-0.

Sen, C. K. and L. Packer. "Antioxidant and redox regulation of gene transcription." *FASEB Journal* 10, no. 7 (maio): 709-20. https://doi.org/10.1096/fasebj.10.7.8635688.

Shkryl, V. M., A. S. Martins, N. D. Ullrich, M. C. Nowycky, E. Niggli and N. Shirokova. 2009. "Reciprocal amplification of ROS and Ca^{2+} signals in stressed mdx dystrophic skeletal muscle fibers." *PflügersArchiv: European Journal of Physiology* 458, no. 5 (setembro): 915-28. https://doi.org/10.1007/s00424-009-0670-2.

Sies, H. and E. Cadenas. 1985. "Oxidative stress: damage to intact cells and organs." *Philosophical Transactions of the Royal Society B: Biological Sciences* 311, no. 1152 (dezembro): 617-31. https://doi.org/10.1098/rstb.1985.0168.

Silva, L. A., P. C. L. Silveira, M. M. Ronsani, P. S. Souza, D. Scheffer e L. C. Vieira. 2011. "Taurine supplementation decreases oxidative stress in skeletal muscle after eccentric exercise." *Cell Biochemistry and Function* 29, no. 1 (janeiro/fevereiro): 43-9. https://doi.org/10.1002/cbf.1716.

Silva, L. A., C. B. Tromm, K. F. Bom, I. Mariano, B. Pozzi, G. L. Rosaet al. 2014. "Effects of taurine supplementation following eccentric exercise in young adults." *Applied Physiology, Nutrition, and Metabolism* 39, no. 1: 101-4. https://doi.org/10.1139/apnm-2012-0229.

Steinbacher, P. and P. Eckl. 2015. "Impact of oxidative stress on exercising skeletal muscle." *Biomolecules* 5, no. 2 (abril): 356-77. https://doi.org/10.3390/biom5020356.

St-Pierre J., J. A. Buckingham, S. J. Roebuck and M. D. Brand. 2002. Topology of superoxide production from different sites in the mitochondrial electron transport chain. *Journal of Biological Chemistry* 277, no. 47 (novembro): 44784-90. https://doi.org/10.1074/jbc.M207217200.

Suchomel, T. J., Nimphius, S., Bellon, C. R., and Stone, M. H. (2018). The importance of muscular strength: training considerations. *Sports medicine*, *48*(4), 765-785.

Talbert, E. E. Smuder, A. J. Min, K. Kwon, O. S. Szeto, H. H. Powers, S. K. 2013. A ativação induzida pela imobilização dos principais sistemas proteolíticos nos músculos esqueléticos é impedida por um antioxidante direcionado às mitocôndrias. *J. Appl. Physiol.* (1985) 115, 529-538. doi: 10.1152/japplphysiol.00471.2013. [Activation induced by the immobilization of the main proteolytic systems in skeletal muscles is prevented by an antioxidant directed at mitochondria]

Thirupathi, A. and R. A. Pinho.2018. "Effects of reactive oxygen species and interplay of antioxidants during physical exercise in skeletal muscles." *Journal of Physiology and Biochemistry* 74, no. 3 (agosto): 359-67. https://doi.org/10.1007/s13105-018-0633-1.

Torres. R., H. J. Appell and J. A. Duarte.2006. "Acute effects of stretching on muscle stiffness after a bout of exhaustive eccentric exercise." *International Journal of Sports Medicine* 28, no. 7: 590-4. https://doi.org/10.1055/s-2007-964865.

Trapp, D., W. Knez and W. Sinclair. 2010. "Could a vegetarian diet reduce exercise-induced oxidative stress? A review of the literature." *Journal of Sports Sciences* 28, no. 12 (outubro): 1261-8. https://doi.org/10.1080/02640414.2010.507676.

Urso, M. L. and P. M. Clarkson.2003. "Oxidative stress, exercise, and antioxidant supplementation." *Toxicology* 189, no. 1-2 (julho): 41-54. https://doi.org/10.1016/S0300-483X(03)00151-3.

Van, L. L. J. Goodpaster, B. H. 2006. "Increased intramuscular lipid storage in the insulin-resistant and endurance-trained state." *PflügersArchiv - European Journal of Physiology* 451, no. 5 (fevereiro): 606-16.https://doi.org/10.1007/s00424-005-1509-0.

Vasilaki, A. and Jackson, M. J. 2013. Papel das espécies reativas de oxigênio na regeneração defeituosa observada no envelhecimento muscular. *Radic livre. Biol. Med.* 65, 317-323. doi: 10.1016/j.freeradbiomed. 2013.07.008.

Vincent, H. K., S. K. Powers, D. J. Stewart, H. A. Demirel, R. A. Shanelyand H. Naito. 2000. "Short-term exercise training improves diaphragm Antioxidant capacity and endurance." *European Journal of Applied Physiology* 81 (janeiro):67-74. https://doi.org/10.1007/PL00013799.

Weineck, J. 2003. *Treinamento ideal.* 9ª ed. São Paulo: Manole.

Whitehead, N. P. Yeung, E. W. Froehner, S. C. Allen, D. G. 2010. A NADPH oxidase do músculo esquelético aumenta e desencadeia danos induzidos por alongamento no mouse mdx. *PLoS ONE* 5: e15354. doi: 10.1371 / journal.pone.0015354. [Skeletal muscle NADPH oxidase increases and triggers stretching-induced damage in the mdx mouse.]

Wright, D. C.; Han, D. H.; Garcia-Roves, P. M.; Geiger, P. C.; Jones, T. E.; J. Holloszy. 2007. "Exercise-induced mitochondrial biogenesis begins before the increase in muscle PGC-1α expression. *Journal of Biological Chemistry* 282 (janeiro): 194-9.https://doi.org/10.1074/jbc.M606116200.

Yan, Z., M. Okutsu, Y. N. Akhtar and V. A. Lira. 2011. "Regulation of exercise-induced fiber type transformation, mitochondrial biogenesis, and angiogenesis in skeletal muscle." *Journal of Applied Physiology* 110, no. 1 (janeiro): 264-74. https://doi.org/10.1152/japplphysiol. 00993.2010.

Yavari, A., M. Javadi, P.Mirmiranand Z. Bahadoran.2015."Exercise-induced oxidative stress and dietary antioxidants." *Asian Journal of Sports Medicine* 6, no. 1 (março):e24898. https://doi.org/ 10.5812/asjsm.24898.

Zuo, L., F. L. Christofi, V. P. Wright, C. Y. Liu, A. J. Merola, L. J. Berliner and T. L. Clanton. 2000. "Intra- and extracellular measurement of reactive oxygen species produced during heat stress in diaphragm muscle." *American Journal of Physiology-Cell Physiology* 279, no. 4 (outubro): C1058-66. https://doi.org/10.1152/ajpcell.2000.279.4.C1058.

BIOGRAPHICAL SKETCHES

Eduardo Borba Neves

Affiliation: Brazilian Army Sports Commission (CDE, Rio de Janeiro, Brazil) and Universidade Tecnológica Federal do Paraná (UTFPR, Curitiba, Brazil)

Education: PhD in Biomedical Engineering

Research and Professional Experience: Eduardo Borba Neves is Colonel of the Brazilian Army, PhD in Biomedical Engineering and PhD in Public Health. He is with the Brazilian Army Sports Commission and with Graduate Program in Biomedical Engineering at the Federal Technological University of Paraná. His major research interests are in the fields of health diagnostic, physical fitness, thermal imaging and therapeutic technologies.

Publications from the Last 3 Years:

Articles in Scientific Journals

1) Fortes García, Rafael Chieza; Melo De Oliveira, Rafael; Martínez, Eduardo Camilo; Borba Neves, Eduardo. VO2 Estimation Equation Accuracy to Young Adults. *Archivos de Medicina* (Manizales), v. 20, p. 33-39, 2020.
2) Lima E Silva, L.; Neves, E.; Silva, J.; Alonso, L.; Vale, R.; Nunes, R.. The haemodynamic demand and the attributes related to the displacement of the soccer referees in the moments of

decision/intervention during the matches. *International Journal of Performance Analysis in Sport,* v. 20, p. 1-12, 2020.

3) Silva, Flávia Da; Yamaguchi, Bruna; Almeida, Karielly Cássia De; Costin, Ana Claudia Martins Szczypior; Maltauro, Luciana; Neves, Eduardo Borba; Mélo, Tainá Ribas. Efeito Imediato, Agudo E Crônico Da Kinesio Taping® Associada À Terapia Neuromotora Intensiva Na Postura Sentada De Crianças Com Paralisia Cerebral. *Arquivos de Ciências da Saúde da UNIPAR,* v. 24, p. 47-52, 2020.

4) Soster Iede Shiguihara, Dryelle; Brandão Oselame, Gleidson; Borba Neves, Eduardo. Tecnologias para o Diagnóstico da Radiodermite: uma Revisão Sistemática. *Archivos de Medicina* (Manizales), v. 20, p. 1-18, 2020. [Technologies for the Diagnosis of Radiodermatitis: a Systematic Review. *Medical Files*]

5) Bernardo, Luciana Dias; Scheeren, Eduardo Mendonça; Marson, Runer Augusto; Neves, Eduardo Borba. Stabilometric changes due to exposure to firearm noise in the Brazilian Army. *Bioscience Journal,* v. 36, p. 1410-1421, 2020.

6) Pucci, G. C. M. F.; Neves, E. B.; Saavedra, F. J. F., Effect of Pilates Method on Physical Fitness Related to Health in the Elderly: A Systematic Review. *Revista Brasileira De Medicina Do Esporte (Online),* v. 25, p. 76-87, 2019. [*Brazilian Journal of Sports Medicine*]

7) Fortes, Marcos De Sá Rego; Rosa, Samir Ezequiel Da; Coutinho, Walmir; Neves, Eduardo Borba. Epidemiological study of metabolic syndrome in Brazilian soldiers. *Archives of Endocrinology Metabolism,* v. 63, p. In Press, 2019.

8) Menegassi, D. A.; Sabbag, Alexandre De Aguiar; Costa, A. R. C.; Maltauro, L.; Mélo, Tainá Ribas; Neves, Eduardo Borba. Terapia neuromotora intensiva melhora a composição corporal na paralisia cerebral e amiotrofia. *Revista Brasileira De Obesidade, Nutrição E Emagrecimento,* v. 13, p. 275-283, 2019. [Intensive neuromotor therapy improves body composition in cerebral palsy and amyotrophy. *Brazilian Journal Of Obesity, Nutrition And Weight Loss*]

9) Lima E. Silva, L.; Godoy, E. S.; Neves, E. B.; Vale, R. G. S.; Lopez, J. A. H.; Nunes, R. A. M.. Heart rate and the distance performed by the soccer referees during matches: a systematic review. *Archivos De Medicina Del Deporte,* v. 36, p. 36-42, 2019.

10) Reis, Victor M.; Neves, Eduardo B.; Garrido, Nuno; Sousa, Ana; Carneiro, André L.; Baldari, Carlo; Barbosa, Tiago. Oxygen Uptake On-Kinetics during Low-Intensity Resistance Exercise: Effect of Exercise Mode and Load. *International Journal of Environmental Research and Public Health,* v. 16, p. 2524, 2019.

11) Magas, Viviane; Abreu De Souza, Mauren; Borba Neves, Eduardo; Nohama, Percy. Evaluation of thermal imaging for the diagnosis of repetitive strain injuries of the wrist and hand joints. *Research on Biomedical Engineering,* v. 35, p. 57-64, 2019.

12) Monteiro, E. R.; Vingren, J.; Correa Neto, V. G.; Neves, E. B; Steele, J.; Novaes, J. S., Effects of Different between Test Rest Intervals in Reproducibility of the 10-Repetition Maximum Load Test: A Pilot Study with Recreationally Resistance Trained Men. *International Journal of Exercise Science,* v. 12, p. 932-940, 2019.

13) Farias, Edvaldo De; Neves, Eduardo Borba; Quaresma, Luis Felgueiras; Vilaça-Alves, José Manuel. Avaliação da qualidade de serviços em Centros de Fitness no Rio de Janeiro: proposta de instrumento específico para instrutores. *Podium: Sport, Leisure and Tourism Review,* v. 8, p. 151-173, 2019. [Evaluation of service quality in Fitness Centers in Rio de Janeiro: proposal for a specific instrument for instructors.]

14) Mélo, Tainá Ribas; Freitas, Jheniffer; Sabbag, Alexandre De Aguiar; Chiarello, Claudiana Renata; Neves, Eduardo Borba; Israel, Vera Lucia. Intensive Neuromotor Therapy improves motor skills of children with Cornelia de Lange Syndrome: case report. *Fisioterapia Em Movimento,* v. 32, p. e003244, 2019.

15) Leal, S. O.; Neves, E. B.; Mello, D. B.; Filgueiras, M. Q.; Dantas, E. M.. Pain perception and thermographic analysis in patients with chronic lower back pain submitted to osteopathic treatment. *Motricidade (Santa Maria Da Feira),* v. 15, p. 12-20, 2019.

16) Neves, E. B. Thermal Imaging in Sports: Athlete's Thermal Passport. *Motricidade (Santa Maria Da Feira)*, v. 15, p. 4-5, 2019.
17) Mélo, Tainá Ribas; Yamaguchi, Bruna; Chiarello, Claudiana Renata; Costin, Ana Cláudia Szczypior; Erthal, Vanessa; Israel, Vera Lúcia; Neves, Eduardo Borba. Intensive neuromotor therapy with suit improves motor gross function in cerebral palsy: a Brazilian study. *Motricidade (Santa Maria Da Feira)*, v. 13, p. 54-61, 2018.
18) Matos, Filipe; Neves, Eduardo Borba; Rosa, Claudio; Reis, Victor Machado; Saavedra, Francisco; Silva, Severiano; Vilaça-Alves, José. Effect of Cold Water Immersion on Elbow Flexors Muscle Thickness after Resistance Training. *Journal of Strength and Conditioning Research*, v. 32, p. 1-763, 2018.
19) Salamunes, Ana Carla Chierighini; Stadnik, Adriana Maria Wan; Neves, Eduardo Borba. Estimation of Female Body Fat Percentage Based on Body Circumferences. *Revista Brasileira De Medicina Do Esporte* (Online), v. 24, p. 97-101, 2018. [Brazilian Journal of Sports Medicine]
20) Santos, Norma Claudia De Macedo Souza; Neves, Eduardo Borba; Fortes, Marcos De Sá Rego; Martinez, Eduardo Camillo; Júnior, Orlando Da Costa Ferreira. The influence of combat simulation exercises on indirect markers of muscle damage in soldiers of the Brazilian army. *Bioscience Journal*, v. 34, p. 1051-1061, 2018.
21) Sabbag, Alexandre De Aguiar; Costin, Ana Claudia Martins Szczypior; Menegassi, Daniel Alves; Silva, Juliana Bertolino; Braga, Marina Marcondes; Neves, Eduardo Borba. Etapa puberal en niños con parálisis cerebral. *Revista Científica General José María Córdova*, v. 16, p. 81-91, 2018. [Pubertal stage in children with cerebral palsy. *General Scientific Journal José María Córdova*]
22) Goncalves, M. M.; Marson, R. A.; Fortes, M. S. R.; Neves, E. B; Rodrigues Neto, G.; Novaes, J. S.. The relationship between handgrip strength and total muscle strength in the Brazilian army military personnel. *Medicina Dello Sport*, v. 71, p. 461-473, 2018.

23) Krueger, E.; Scheeren, E. M.; Rinaldin, C. D. P.; Lazzaretti, A. E.; Neves, E. B; Nogueira Neto, G. N.; Nohama, P. Impact of Skinfold Thickness on Wavelet-Based Mechanomyographic Signal. *Facta Universitatis,* v. 16, p. 359-368, 2018.

24) Oliveira, M. C. N.; Melo, T. R.; Pol, Stéphani; Costin, Ana Claudia Martins Szczypior; Oliveira, F. C. N.; Neves, E. B. Terapia neuromotora intensiva promove ganhos de habilidades motoras grossas e manutenção da composição corporal em crianças com paralisia cerebral. *Revista Brasileira De Obesidade, Nutrição E Emagrecimento,* v. 12, p. 598-606, 2018. [Intensive neuromotor therapy promotes gains in gross motor skills and maintenance of body composition in children with cerebral palsy. *Brazilian Journal Of Obesity, Nutrition And Weight Loss*]

25) Uchôa, Paulo; Matos, Filipe; Neves, Eduardo Borba; Saavedra, Francisco; Rosa, Claudio; Reis, Victor Machado; Vilaça-Alves, José. Evaluation of two different resistance training volumes on the skin surface temperature of the elbow flexors assessed by thermography. *Infrared Physics & Technology,* v. 93, p. 178-183, 2018.

26) Neves, E. B.; Garcia, Rafael Chieza Fortes; De Oliveira, Rafael Melo; Martinez, Eduardo Camillo. Incidence rate of musculoskeletal injuries in Brazilian army. *Bioscience Journal,* p. 1744-1750, 2018.

27) Santos, L. C.; Cherem, E. H.; Azeredo, F. P.; Neves, E. B; Oliveira, D. R.; Novaes, G. S.; Silva, A. J.; Novaes, J. S.. Effects of different strength training programs in young males maximal strength and anthropometrics. *Motricidade (Santa Maria Da Feira),* v. 14, p. 301-309, 2018.

28) Welter, D. L.; Neves, E. B.; Saavedra, F. J. F., Profile of practitioners of supervised physical exercise in the Southern region of Brazil. *Bioscience Journal* (UFU), v. 33, p. 209-218, 2017.

29) Sumini, K. L.; Oselame, G. B.; Oselame, C. S.; Dutra, Denecir De Almeida; Neves, E. B. Alimentação, risco cardiovascular e nível de atividade física em adolescentes. *Revista Brasileira de Obesidade,*

Nutrição e Emagrecimento, v. 11, p. 23-30, 2017. [Diet, cardiovascular risk and physical activity level in adolescents. *Brazilian Journal of Obesity, Nutrition and Weight Loss*]

30) Salamunes, Ana Carla Chierighini; Stadnik, Adriana Maria Wan; Neves, Eduardo Borba. The effect of body fat percentage and body fat distribution on skin surface temperature with infrared thermography. *Journal of Thermal Biology*, v. 66, p. 1-9, 2017.

31) Garrett, Camylla Aparecida; Oselame, Gleidson Brandão; Neves, Eduardo Borba. O uso da episiotomia no Sistema Único de Saúde Brasileiro: a percepção das parturientes. *Revista Saúde e Pesquisa*, v. 9, p. 453-459, 2017. [The use of episiotomy in the Brazilian Unified Health System: the perception of parturients. *Health and Research Magazine*]

32) Oselame, Gleidson Brandão; Sanches, Ionildo José; Kuntze, Alana; Neves, Eduardo Borba. Software for automatic diagnostic prediction of skin clinical images based on ABCD rule. *Bioscience Journal*, v. 33, p. 1065-1078, 2017.

33) Crivellaro, Jackeline; Almeida, Renan Moritz Varnier Rodrigues De; Wenke, Rodney; Neves, Eduardo Borba. Perfil De Lesões Em Pilotos De Parapente No Brasil E Seus Fatores De Risco. *Revista Brasileira de Medicina do Esporte*, v. 23, p. 270-273, 2017. [Profile of Injuries in Paragliding Pilots in Brazil and Their Risk Factors. *Brazilian Journal of Sports Medicine*]

34) Goncalves, M. M.; Marson, R. A.; Fortes, M. S. R.; Neves, E. B.; Novaes, J. S., The relationship between total muscle strength and anthropometric indicators in Brazilian Army military. *Revista Brasileira De Obesidade, Nutrição E Emagrecimento*, V. 11, p. 330-337, 2017. [The relationship between total muscle strength and anthropometric indicators in Brazilian Army military. *Brazilian Journal Of Obesity, Nutrition And Weight Loss*]

35) Melo De Oliveira, Rafael; Carreiro Lermen, Daniel; Augusto Marson, Runer; Borba Neves, Eduardo. La influencia del calentamiento activo, con o sin estiramiento estático, sobre la fuerza muscular en militares brasileños. *Revista Científica General José*

María Córdova, v. 15, p. 157-166, 2017. [The influence of active warm-up, with or without static stretching, on muscular strength in Brazilian military personnel. *General Scientific Journal José María Córdova*]

36) Santos, Michele Caroline Dos; Krueger, Eddy; Neves, Eduardo Borba. Electromyographic analysis of postural overload caused by bulletproof vests on public security professionals. *Research on Biomedical Engineering*, v. 33, p. 175-184, 2017.

37) De Souza, Rodrigo Poderoso; Cirilo De Sousa, Maria Do Socorro; Neves, Eduardo Borba; Rosa, Claudio; Cruz, Igor Raineh Durães; Targino Júnior, Adenilson; Macedo, José Onaldo Ribeiro; Reis, Victor Machado; Vilaça-Alves, José. Acute effect of a fight of Mixed Martial Arts (MMA) on the serum concentrations of testosterone, cortisol, creatine kinase, lactate, and glucose. *Motricidade (Santa Maria Da Feira)*, v. 13, p. 30-37, 2017.

38) Ulbrich, G. D. S.; Oselame, Gleidson Brandão; Oliveira, E. M.; Neves, E. B. Motivadores da ideação suicida e a autoagressão em adolescentes. *Adolescência & Saúde*, v. 14, p. 40-46, 2017. [Motivators of suicidal ideation and self-harm in adolescents. *Adolescence & Health*]

39) Neves, Eduardo Borba; Salamunes, Ana Carla Chierighini; De Oliveira, Rafael Melo; Stadnik, Adriana Maria Wan. Effect of body fat and gender on body temperature distribution. *Journal of Thermal Biology*, v. 70, p. 1-8, 2017.

40) Neves, Eduardo Borba; Eraso, Natalia Morales; Narváez, Yesenia Seña; Rairan, Fabian Steven Garay; Garcia, Rafael Chieza Fortes. Musculoskeletal Injuries in sergeants training courses from Brazil and Colombia. *Journal of Science and Medicine in Sport*, v. 20, p. S117, 2017.

41) Neves, Eduardo Borba. Physical fitness tests in Latin American Armies. *Journal of Science and Medicine in Sport*, v. 20, p. S60, 2017.

42) Neves, Eduardo Borba; Da Rosa, Samir Ezequiel; Fortes, Marcos De Sá Rego. Prevalence and anthropometric predictors of metabolic

syndrome in the Brazilian military. *Journal of Science and Medicine in Sport,* v. 20, p. S158, 2017.
43) Neves, Eduardo Borba; Rouboa, Abel; Machado, Leandro. Technologies for Assessment of Training Effects on Health and Performance. *The Open Sports Sciences Journal,* v. 10, p. 222-222, 2017.
44) Capitani, Gabriel; Sehnem, Eduardo; Rosa, Claudio; Matos, Filipe; Reis, Victor M.; Neves, Eduardo B.. Osgood-schlatter Disease Diagnosis by Algometry and Infrared Thermography. *The Open Sports Sciences Journal,* v. 10, p. 223-228, 2017.
45) Oselame, Cristiane Da Silva; Oselame, Gleidson Brandão; De Matos, Oslei; Neves, Eduardo Borba. Equation to Fat Percentage Estimation in Women with Reduced Bone Mineral Density. *The Open Sports Sciences Journal,* v. 10, p. 251-256, 2017.
46) Zaar, Andrigo; Neves, Eduardo Borba; Rouboa, Abel Ilah; Reis, Victor Machado. Determinative Factors in the Injury Incidence on Runners: Synthesis of Evidence -Injuries on Runners-. *The Open Sports Sciences Journal,* v. 10, p. 294-304, 2017.
47) Neves, Eduardo Borba. Correlations between the simulated military tasks performance and physical fitness tests at high altitude. *Motricidade (Santa Maria Da Feira),* v. 13, p. 12-17, 2017.

Danielli Braga de Mello

Affiliation: Physical Education College of Brazilian Army (EsEFEx, EB, RJ, Brazil)

Education: Graduation in Physical Education Federal at University of Rio de Janeiro (UFRJ, RJ, Brazil); Master in Human Kinetics Science at Castelo Branco University (UCB, RJ, Brazil); PhD in Public Health at Oswaldo Cruz Foundation (FIOCRUZ, RJ, Brazil), Post-Doctorate in Extreme Environmental Physiology at University of Portsmouth, UK, Post-

Doctorate in Thermography applied to Sport at Universidad Politecnica de Madrid, Spain.

Research Experience: Physiology of Exercise.

Professional Experience: Lecture (under graduation and Post-graduation), Coordination and Research. Associate professor at EsEFEx, collaborating professor of the *stricto sensu* program in exercise and sport sciences (PPGCEE) at State University of Rio de Janeiro (UERJ), collaborating professor of the *stricto sensu* program in Biosciences of Human Motricity at Federal State University of Rio de Janeiro (UNIRIO), Adjunct Editor-in-Chief of the Journal of Physical Education (REF / JPE), author of the book indoor cycling.

Publications from the Last 3 Years:

Articles in Scientific Journals

1) Mello, T. F.; Fortes, M. S. R.; Mello, D. B.; Rosa, G. Análise da concordância entre diferentes índices de composição corporal em estudantes do sexo feminino. *Adolescência & Saúde.* v.17, p.99 - 105, 2020. [Analysis of the agreement between different body composition indexes in female students. *Adolescence & Health*]
2) Szpilman, D.; Mello, Danielli Braga de; Queiroga, A. C.; Ferreira, Rogério Emygdio. Association of Drowning Mortality with Preventive Interventions: A Quarter of a Million Deaths Evaluation in Brazil. *International Journal of Aquatic Research and Education,* v.12, p.3 - 1, 2020.
3) Oliveira Leal, S. M.; Neves, E. B.; Mello, D. B.; Filgueiras, M. Q.; Dantas, E. H. M. Pain perception and thermographic analysis in patients with chronic lower back pain submitted to osteopathic treatment. *Motricidade (Santa Maria Da Feira).* v.15, p.12 - 20, 2020.
4) Dias Henriques, Ighor Amadeu; Braga De Mello, Danielli; Ribeiro

Filho, Kennedy Car; Brandão Pinto De Castro, Juliana; Gomes De Souza Vale, Rodrigo; Rosa, Guilherme. Respuestas de la presión arterial en individuos normotensos sometidos a diferentes intensidades en sesiones de entrenamiento de fuerza. *Revista De Ciencias De La Actividad Física.* v.21, p.1 - 13, 2020. [Blood pressure responses in normotensive individuals subjected to different intensities in strength training sessions. *Journal of Physical Activity Sciences*]

5) Della Corte, J.; Rangel, L.; Vale, R. G. S.; Danielli Braga De Mello; Pardo, Pjm; Rosa, G. ¿Afecta el entrenamento intervalado de alta intensidad (HIIT) al desempeño en el entrenamento de la fuerza? *Archivos De Medicina Del Deporte,* v.36, p.8 - 12, 2019. [Does High Intensity Interval Training (HIIT) Affect Strength Training Performance? *Sports Medicine Archives*]

6) Schaly, D.; Rosa, G; Fin, G.; Mello, D. B.; Baretta, E.; Jesus, J. A.; Nodari Junior, R. J. Composição corporal e aptidão cardiorrespiratória de escolares do Meio Oeste de Santa Catarina. *Revista Brasileira De Obesidade, Nutrição E Emagrecimento.* v.13, p.21 - 27, 2019. [Body composition and cardiorespiratory fitness of schoolchildren from the Midwest of Santa Catarina. Brazilian *Journal Of Obesity, Nutrition And Weight Loss*]

7) Nogueira, C. J.; Galdino, L. A. S.; Cortez, A. C. L.; Souza, I. V.; Mello, Danielli Braga De; Senna, G. W.; Brandao, P. P.; Dantas, Estélio H. M. Effects of flexibility training with different volumes and intensities on the vertical jump performance of adult women. *Journal Of Physical Education And Sport,* v.19, p.1680 - 1685, 2019.

8) Monteiro-Lago, T.; Cardoso, M. S.; Henriques, I.; Mello, D. B.; Fortes, Marcos de Sá R.; Vale, R. G. S.; Rosa, Guilherme. Impact of eight weeks of concurrent training on obesity-related biochemical parameters and cardiometabolic risk factors: a case report. *Obesity, Weight Managment & Control,* v.1, p.98 - 103, 2019.

9) Szpilman, D.; Mello, Danielli Braga. Recomendações SOBRASA: "Checklist" individual do atleta para reduzir eventos adversos em

águas abertas. *Revista de Educação Física/Journal of Physical Education*, v.88, p.1034 - 1040, 2019. [SOBRASA Recommendations: Individual athlete's checklist to reduce adverse events in open water. *Journal of Physical Education / Journal of Physical Education*]

10) Rosa, Guilherme; Henriques, Ighor; Soutinho, Ingrid De Freitas; Silva, Gustavo Neves Monteiro; Mello, Danielli Braga De; Pereira, Fábio Dutra. Respostas Fisiológicas Ao Exercício Aquático Em Gestantes Hipertensa E Normotensa: Relato De Caso Controle. *Revista de Investigación en Actividades Acuáticas*, v.3, p.14 - 17, 2019. [Physiological Responses to Aquatic Exercise in Hypertensive and Normotensive Pregnant Women: Case Control Report. *Journal of Research in Aquatic Activities*]

11) Mello, Danielli Braga. Estresse Térmico – os efeitos do calor sobre o desempenho físico. *Revista de Educação Física - Escola de Educação Física do Exército*, v.87, p.541 - 545, 2018. [Thermal Stress - the effects of heat on physical performance. *Revista de Educação Fisica - Army Physical Education School*]

12) Granja, E.; Pinto, E. M. M.; Reis, A. O.; Mello, D. B.; Rosa, G. Hemodynamics in resistance training: a comparative analysis between multi and single-joint exercises. *Medicina Dello Sport*, v.71, p.514 - 520, 2018.

13) Vieira, L.; Faria Jr., A. G.; Mello, D. B.; Santos, R. F.; Martins, L. C. X.; Capinussú, J. M. Política nacional para a detecção de talentos esportivos: uma proposta baseada em experiências de sucesso. *Revista de Educação Física - Escola de Educação Física do Exército*, v.87, p.461 - 471, 2018. [National policy for the detection of sports talents: a proposal based on successful experiences. *Revista de Educação Fisica - Army Physical Education School*]

14) Santos, D. F.; Diniz, M. L.; Cardoso, G. A.; Mello, D. B.; Vale, R. G. S.; Dantas, E. H. M. Autonomia funcional de idosas fisicamente ativas e insuficientemente ativas de uma cidade do centro sul cearense: um estudo seccional. *Revista de Educação Física*, v.86, p.250 - 255, 2017. [Functional autonomy of physically active and

insufficiently active elderly women in a city in the south of Ceará: a sectional study. *Physical Education Magazine*]

15) Silva, R. C. F.; Pereira, F. D.; Mello, D. B.; Alias, A.; Rosa, G. Efectos agudos del ciclismo indoor en la presión inspiratoria máxima (PIMax) y la presión espiratoria máxima (PEMax) de adultos activos. *Revista De Ciencias De La Actividad Física*, v.18, p.25 - 31, 2017. [Acute effects of indoor cycling on peak inspiratory pressure (PIMax) and peak expiratory pressure (PEMax) of active adults. *Journal of Physical Activity Sciences*]

16) Sodre, R. S.; Soares, R. P. S.; Silva, G. P.; Fonseca, T. M.; Mello, D. B.; Rosa, G. Efeitos de 12 meses de hidroginástica sobre o estado nutricional, pressão arterial de repouso e dosagem medicamentosa de idosas hipertensas. *Revista de Investigación en Actividades Acuáticas*, v.1, p.45 - 48, 2017. [Effects of 12 months of aqua aerobics on nutritional status, resting blood pressure and medication dosage of elderly hypertensive women. *Revista de Investigación en Acuáticas Activities*]

17) Quintão Coelho Rocha, Cristiano Andrade; Guimarães, Andrea Carmen; Borba'pinheiro, Claudio Joaquim; Santos, César Augusto De Souza; Moreira, Maria Helena Rodrigues; Mello, Danielli Braga de; Dantas, Estélio Henrique Martin. Efeitos de 20 semanas de treinamento combinado na capacidade funcional de idosas. *Revista Brasileira De Ciências Do Esporte*, v.39, p.442 - 449, 2017. [Effects of 20 weeks of combined training on the functional capacity of elderly women. *Brazilian Journal of Sport Sciences*]

18) Santana, T. C.; Mello, Danielli Braga de; Maia Jr., J. M. M.; Mainenti, M. Nível de hidratação e reposição hídrica dos atletas da seleção brasileira militar de futebol: comportamento semelhante nas diferentes posições da equipe. *Revista Brasileira De Futebol*, v.8, p.24 - 35, 2017. [Hydration level and water replacement of athletes from the Brazilian military football team: similar behavior in the different positions of the team. *Brazilian Football Magazine*]

Books

1) Mello, Danielli Braga de. *Ciclismo indoor: bases científicas e metodológicas.* São Paulo: RV Editorial, 2020, v.1000. p.248. [*Indoor cycling: scientific and methodological bases.*]
2) Mello, D. B. *Ciclismo Indoor - Bases Científicas e Metodológicas.* Rio de Janeiro: Sprint, 2004. [*Indoor Cycling - Scientific and Methodological Bases.*]

Book's Chapters

1) Mello, Danielli B.; Cader, S. A.; Pernambuco, C. S.; Vale, R. G. S.; Dantas, E. H. M. Bases de entrenamiento deportivo para adultos mayores: procedimientos de evaluación In: *Evaluación de la calidad de vida, cognición, depresióm, autoestima y autoimagen.* 1 ed. Madrid: Dykinson SL, 2019, v.1, p. 145-172. [Bases of sports training for older adults: evaluation procedures In: *Evaluation of quality of life, cognition, depression, self-esteem and self-image*]
2) Alias, A.; Mello, D. B. Termorregulación en deportistas paralímpicos In: *Aplicaciones de intervención en actividade física adaptada.* 1 ed. Madrid: Dykinson S. L., 2019, v.1, p. 63-74. [Thermoregulation in Paralympic athletes In: *Intervention applications in adapted physical activity.*]
3) Barneche, T. F.; Mello, D. B.; Alias, A. G.; Pinheiro, J. G.; Stocchero, C. A. Efeitos do Tai Chi Chuan e Yoga sobre a densidade mineral óssea: uma revisão sistemática In: *VI Congreso Internacional de Deporte Inclusivo.* 1 ed. Almería: Universidad de Almería, 2017, p. 145-153. [Effects of Tai Chi Chuan and Yoga on bone mineral density: a systematic review In: *VI Congreso Internacional de Deporte Inclusivo.*]
4) Vale, R. G. S.; Rosa, Guilherme; Mello, Danielli Braga de; Pardo, P. J. M.; Dantas, E. H. M. Strength exercise and cardiometabolic health In: *Advances in Medicine and Biology.* 1 ed. New York: Nova Medical, 2017, v.1, p. 59-82.

Rogério Santo de Aguiar

Affiliation: Laboratório do Exercício e do Esporte (LABEES), Programa de Pós-Graduação em Ciências do Exercício e do Esporte (PPGCEE), Universidade do Estado do Rio de Janeiro (UERJ)

Education: PhD student at the Post-Graduate Program in Exercise and Sport Sciences, Rio de Janeiro State University, RJ, Brazil. Master of Science in Human Motricity. Castelo Branco University. RJ, Brazil. Post graduate in Science of Physical Preparation. Castelo Branco University. RJ, Brazil. Graduated in Physical Education. Castelo Branco University. RJ, Brazil.

Research and Professional Experience: Researcher by Laboratory of Exercise and Sport, Rio de Janeiro State University, RJ, Brazil. He was Professor of Graduation at Castelo Branco University (CBU), RJ, Brazil, in the discipline Methods of training of bodybuilding I and II. He was professor and advisor of the master's in the discipline Research Methodology CBU, RJ, Brazil. He received a scholarship from the Research Support Foundation of the State of Rio de Janeiro (FAPERJ), in the project: Elaboration of a Nutritional supplements in gel Containing Açaí Microcapsules and its use in Individuals Trained to Reduce Oxidative Stress. He has experience in Physical Education and Health, with an emphasis on Physical Conditioning, Strength Training, Biomechanics and Exercise Physiology, Musculoskeletal Rehabilitation, Oxidative Stress and Quality of Life. He is a researcher on topics on: Electromyography, Thermography, Strength Training, Oxidative Stress, Hormones, Muscle Fatigue and Quality of Life.

Publications from the Last 3 Years:

Articles in Scientific Journals

1) Juliana B. P. de Castro; Rodrigo G. de S. Vale; Aguiar, Rogério Santos; Rafael da Silva Mattos. Perfil do estilo de vida de

universitários de Educação Física da cidade do Rio de Janeiro. *Revista Brasileira de Ciência e Movimento*, v. 25, p. 73-83, 2017. [Lifestyle profile of Physical Education students in the city of Rio de Janeiro. *Brazilian Journal of Science and Movement*]

2) Juliana Brandão Pinto de Castro, Rogério Santos de Aguiar, Gabriela Rezende de Oliveira Venturini, Andressa Oliveira Barros dos Santos, Glória de Paula Silva, Tainah de Paula Lima, Vitor Ayres Principe, Rodrigo Gomes de Souza Vale. The Effects of Physical Exercise on Insulin-Like Growth Factor I in Older Women: A Systematic Review. *Journal of Exercise Physiology online.* v. 22, n. 7, 2019.

Book chapters:

1) Vale, R. G. S.; Silva, J. B.; Aguiar, R. S.; Castro, J. B. P.; Borba-Pinheiro, Claudio Joaquim. Exame físico no idoso In: *Aspectos biopsicossociais do envelhecimento e a prevenção de quedas na terceira idade.* 1 ed. Joaçaba, SC: Editora Unoesc, 2017, v.1, p. 71-112. ISBN: 9788584221455. [Physical examination in the elderly In: *Biopsychosocial aspects of aging and the prevention of falls in old age.*]

Juliana Brandão Pinto de Castro

Affiliation: Laboratório do Exercício e do Esporte (LABEES), Universidade do Estado do Rio de Janeiro (UERJ)

Education: PhD in Exercise and Sports Sciences

Research and Professional Experience: Physical Education

Publications from the Last 3 Years:

Articles in Scientific Journals

1) Matos, F. P.; Dantas, E. H. M.; Oliveira, F. B.; Castro, J. B. P.; Conceiçâo, M. C. S. C.; Nunes, R. A. M.; Vale, R. G. S. Analysis of the pain symptoms, flexibility, and hydroxyproline concentration in individuals with low back pain submitted to Global Postural Re-education and stretching. *Pain Management,* v.10, p.167 - 177, 2020.
2) Castro, J. B. P.; Lima, V. P.; Santos, A. O. B.; Silva, G. C. P. S. M.; Oliveira, J. G. M.; Silva, J. N. L.; Vale, R. G. S. Correlation analysis between biochemical markers, pain perception, low back functional disability, and muscle strength in postmenopausal women with low back pain. *Journal of Physical Education and Sport,* v.20, p.24 - 30, 2020.
3) Della Corte, J.; Pereira, W. L. M.; Corrêa, E. E. L. S.; Oliveira, J. G. M.; Lima, B. L. P.; Castro, J. B. P.; Lima, V. P. Influence of power and maximal strength training on thermal reaction and vertical jump performance in Brazilian basketball players: a preliminary study. *Biomedical Human Kinetics,* v.12, p.91 - 100, 2020.
4) Paz, G. A.; Maia, M. F.; Miranda, H.; Castro, J. B. P.; Willardson, J. M. Maximal strength performance, efficiency, and myoelectric responses with differing intra-set rest intervals during paired set training. *Journal of Bodywork and Movement Therapies,* v.24, p.263 - 268, 2020.
5) Henriques, I. A. D.; Mello, D. B.; Ribeiro Filho, K. C.; Castro, J. B. P.; Vale, R. G. S.; Rosa, G. Respostas pressóricas em indivíduos normotensos submetidos a diferentes intensidades em sessões de treinamento de força. *Revista De Ciencias De La Actividad Física,* v.21, p.1 - 13, 2020. [Pressure responses in normotensive individuals submitted to different intensities in strength training sessions]

6) Castro, J. B. P.; Brum, R. D. O.; Pernambuco, C. S.; Vale, R. G. S. Análise De Correlação Entre Força Muscular, Igf-1 E Autonomia Funcional Em Idosas Com Excesso De Peso Submetidas A Exercícios Resistidos Aquáticos. *Revista de Investigación en Actividades Acuáticas,* v.3, p.18 - 23, 2019. [Correlation Analysis Between Muscular Strength, Igf-1 And Functional Autonomy In Overweight Elderly Women Undergoing Aquatic Resistance Exercises.]
7) Gama, D. R. N.; Nunes, R. A. M.; Castro, J. B. P.; Souza, C. A. M.; Rodrigues Júnior, F. L.; Vale, R. G. S. *Analysis of the relationship between personality traits and leadership characteristics of handball coaches of school teams in the state of Rio de Janeiro, Brazil.* Motriz, v.25, p.e101925, 2019.
8) Leite Junior, O. D.; Vale, R. G. S.; Castro, J. B. P.; Oliveira, F. B.; Gama, D. R. N.; Oliveira Filho, G. R.; Fonseca, B. B.; Reis, V. M. M. R.; Nunes, R. A. M. Cardiorespiratory responses in maximal cycle ergometry in cardiac rehabilitation. *Journal of Physical Education and Sport,* v.19, p.393 - 404, 2019.
9) Venturini, G. R. O.; Silva, N. S. L.; Almada, L. B.; Castro, J. B. P.; Mazini Filho, M. L.; Vale, R. G. S. Comparação entre indicadores de saúde de alunos do ensino médio das redes federal, estadual e particular de Minas Gerais, Brasil. *Motricidade (Santa Maria Da Feira),* v.15, p.87 - 95, 2019. [Comparison between health indicators of high school students from federal, state and private schools in Minas Gerais, Brazil. *Motricity (Santa Maria Da Feira)*]
10) Lima, B. L. P.; Leopoldo Junior, M. N.; Santos, T. L. R.; Silva, J. B.; Nunes, R. A. M.; Vale, R. G. S.; Castro, J. B. P.; Lima, V. P. Comparación del perfil antropométrico y la aptitud física de los atletas de baloncesto de diferentes posiciones. *Revista De Ciencias De La Actividad Física,* v.20, p.1 - 13, 2019. [Comparison of the anthropometric profile and physical fitness of basketball athletes of different positions. *Journal of Physical Activity Sciences*]
11) Pernambuco, C. S.; Lima, J. O.; Cortez, A. C. L.; Castro, J. B. P.; Vale, R. G. S.; Oliveira, C. C. C.; Dantas, E. H. M. Effects of

electroacupuncture on body mass index and quality of life of nurses from Gaffrée and Guinle University Hospital. *International Journal of Development Research,* v.9, p.25398 - 25402, 2019.

12) Machado, A. F.; Castro, J. B. P.; Bocalini, D. S.; Figueira Junior, A. J.; Nunes, R. A. M.; Vale, R. G. S. Effects of plyometric training on the performance of 5-km road runners. *Journal of Physical Education and Sport,* v.19, p.691 - 695, 2019.

13) Mattos, R. S.; Castro, J. B. P.; Sabino, C.; Espírito Santo, W. R.; Florentino, J. O.; Menezes, L. S.; Oliveira, L. H. S.; Nascimento, S. S. O mito contemporâneo da heroína esportiva: da guerra ao pódio. *Caderno De Educação Física E Esporte,* v.17, p.1 - 8, 2019.

14) Paz, G. A.; Maia, M. F.; Sant'ana, H. G.; Miranda, H.; Castro, J. B. P.; Lima, V. P. Positional relationship between several performance tests and physical profile of Brazilian football athletes. *Acta Scientiarum. Health Sciences (Online),* v.41, p.43155 -, 2019.

15) Mattos, Rafael Da Silva; Grivet, Eliane De Queiroz; Castro, Juliana Brandão Pinto De; Espírito Santo, Wecisley Ribeiro do; Sabino, César; Retondar, Jeferson José Moebus; GAMA, Dirceu Ribeiro Nogueira da. Sobrevivendo ao estigma da hipertrofia: notas etnográficas sobre o fisiculturismo feminino. *Arquivos Em Movimento (Ufrj. Online),* v.15, p.97 - 113, 2019. [Dirceu Ribeiro Nogueira da. Surviving the stigma of hypertrophy: ethnographic notes on female bodybuilding. *Moving Files* (Ufrj. Online)]

16) Castro, J. B. P.; Aguiar, R. S.; Venturini, G. R. O.; Santos, A. O. B.; Silva, G. P.; Lima, T. P.; Principe, V. A.; Vale, R. G. S. The effects of physical exercise on insulin-like growth factor I in older women: a systematic review. *Journal of Exercise Physiology Online,* v.22, p.88 - 99, 2019.

17) Della Corte, J.; Pinheiro, C. B.; Lima, B. L. P.; Vignoli, F. A.; Oliveira, J. G. M.; Castro, J. B. P.; Lima, V. P. Thermographic analysis of thighs of trained men during the leg extension exercise. *Journal of Physical Education and Sport,* v.19, p.2458 - 2465, 2019.

18) Silva, L. L.; Martins, L. C. X.; Gama, D. R. N.; Castro, J. B. P.; Godoy, E. S.; Nunes, R. A. M. Análise Da Relação Entre

Competência Técnica E Intenções Morais Em Tomadas De Decisão De Árbitros De Futebol: Um Estudo Exploratório Com Crianças. *Pensar A Prática* (Ufg. Impresso), v.21, p.598 - 608, 2018. [Analysis of the Relationship between Technical Competence and Moral Intentions in Decision Making by Soccer Referees: An Exploratory Study with Children. *Thinking Practice* (Ufg. Printed)]

19) Castro, Juliana Brandão Pinto de; Vale, Rodrigo Gomes de Souza; Chame, Flávio; Benittez, Hugo Seixas Pinto Azevedo; SILVA, Jurandir Baptista da; Nunes, Rodolfo de Alkmim Moreira; Mattos, Rafael da Silva Análise de conhecimentos e hábitos de hidratação de corredores de rua no município do Rio de Janeiro. *Revista Brasileira De Prescrição E Fisiologia Do Exercício*, v.12, p.339 - 348, 2018. [Analysis of knowledge and hydration habits of street runners in the city of Rio de Janeiro. *Brazilian Journal of Prescription and Exercise Physiology*]

20) Venturini, G. R. O.; Mazini Filho, M. L.; Touguinha, H. M.; Castro, J. B. P.; Pereira, M. R.; Vale, R. G. S. Análise do conceito de saúde abordado nas aulas de Educação Física escolar: uma revisão integrativa. *Revista Interdisciplinar de Promoção da Saúde*, v.1, p.119 - 126, 2018. [Analysis of the health concept covered in school Physical Education classes: an integrative review. *Interdisciplinary Journal of Health Promotion*]

21) Vale, Rodrigo Gomes de Souza; Castro, Juliana Brandão Pinto de; Mattos, Rafael da Silva; Rodrigues, Vanessa Ferreira; Oliveira, Flávio Boechat de; GAMA, Dirceu Ribeiro Nogueira da; ROSA, Guilherme; Nunes, Rodolfo de Alkmim Moreira. Analysis of balance, muscle strength, functional autonomy, and quality of life in elderly women submitted to a strength and walking program. *Journal of Exercise Physiology Online*, v.21, p.13 - 24, 2018.

22) Silva, J. B.; Lima, V. P.; Castro, J. B. P.; Paz, G. A.; Novaes, J. S.; Nunes, R. A. M.; Vale, R. G. S. Analysis of myoelectric activity, blood lactate concentration and time under tension in repetitions maximum in the squat exercise. *Journal of Physical Education and Sport*, v.18, p.2478 - 2485, 2018.

23) Gama, D. R. N.; Nunes, R. A. M.; Guimarães, G. L.; Silva, L. L.; Castro, J. B. P.; Vale, R. G. S. Analysis of the burnout levels of soccer referees working at amateur and professional leagues of Rio de Janeiro, Brazil. *Journal Of Physical Education And Sport,* v.18, p.1168 - 1174, 2018.

24) Santos, D. T. N.; Mendes, L. T.; Alves, M. F. N.; Bonela, A. C. C.; Paz, G. A.; Silva, J. B.; Castro, J. B. P.; Batista, C. A. S.; Sant'ana, H. G.; Lima, V. P.; Miranda, H. L. Comparison of different flexibility training methods and specific warm-up on repetition maximum volume in lower limb exercises with female jazz dancers. *Journal of Human Sport and Exercise,* v.13, p.18 - 28, 2018.

25) Salarolli, L. C. W.; Barros, R. M. B.; Silva, J. B.; Carvalho, I. L. S.; Vale, R. G. S.; Nunes, R. A. M.; Castro, J. B. P.; Lima, V. P. Comparison of time under tension, repetition maximum and electromyographic activity in bench press exercise in different speeds execution. *Gazzetta Medica Italiana. Archivio Per Le Scienze Mediche (Testo Stampato),* v.177, p.637 - 644, 2018.

26) Mazini Filho, Mauro Lúcio; Savoia, Rafael Pedroza; Castro, Juliana Brandão Pinto De; Moreira, Osvaldo Costa; Venturini, Gabriela Rezende De Oliveira; Curty, Victor Magalhães; Ferreira, Maria Elisa Caputo. Effects of hypnotic induction on muscular strength in men with experience in resistance training. *Journal of Exercise Physiology Online,* v.21, p.52 - 61, 2018.

27) Vale, R. G. S.; Gama, D. R. N.; Oliveira, F. B.; Almeida, D. S. M.; Castro, J. B. P.; Alarcon Meza, E. I.; Mattos, R. S.; Nunes, R. A. M. Effects of resistance training and chess playing on the quality of life and cognitive performance of elderly women: a randomized controlled trial. *Journal of Physical Education and Sport.,* v.18, p.1469 - 1477, 2018.

28) Raymundo, A. C. G.; Pernambuco, C. S.; Brum, R. D. O.; Castro, J. B. P.; Oliveira, F. B.; Gama, D. R. N.; Nunes, R. A. M.; Vale, R. G. S. Evaluation of strength, agility and aerobic capacity in Brazilian football players. *Biomedical Human Kinetics,* v.10, p.25 - 30, 2018.

29) Mazini Filho, Mauro Lúcio; Venturini, Gabriela Rezende De Oliveira; Castro, Juliana Brandão Pinto De; Silveira, Alessandra Rodrigues Da; Souza, Rodrigo Marçal De; Mantovani Neto, José; Ferreira, Maria Elisa Caputo. Força e potência muscular para autonomia funcional de idosos: uma breve revisão narrativa. *Revista de Educação Física - Escola de Educação Física do Exército,* v.87, p.439 - 446, 2018. [Muscle strength and power for functional autonomy in the elderly: a brief narrative review. *Revista de Educação Fisica - Army Physical Education School*]

30) Della Corte, J.; Paz, G. A.; Castro, J. B. P.; Miranda, H. Hypotensive effect induced by strength training using the DeLorme and Oxford methods in trained men. *Polish Journal of Sport and Tourism,* v.25, p.23 - 30, 2018.

31) Souza, Anna Carolina Carvalho De; Mattos, Rafael Da Silva; Castro, Juliana Brandão Pinto De; Retondar, Jeferson José Moebus. O desenvolvimento socioafetivo da criança: influências do profissional de Educação Física. *Coleção Pesquisa Em Educação Física,* v.17, p.95 - 102, 2018. [The child's socio-affective development: influences of the Physical Education professional. *Physical Education Research Collection*]

32) Lima, V. P.; Nunes, R. A. M.; Silva, J. B.; Paz, G. A.; Jesus, M.; Castro, J. B. P.; Dantas, E. H. M.; Vale, R. G. S. Pain perception and low back pain functional disability after a 10-week core and mobility training program: A pilot study. *Journal of Back and Musculoskeletal Rehabilitation,* v.31, p.637 - 643, 2018.

33) Gama, D. R. N.; Barreto, H. D.; Castro, J. B. P.; Nunes, R. A. M.; Vale, R. G. S. Relationships between personality traits and resilience levels of jiu-jitsu and kickboxing Brazilian athletes. *Archives of Budo Science of Martial Arts and Extreme Sports,* v.14, p.125 - 133, 2018.

34) Oliveira, Lucas Silva Franco De; Mazini Filho, Mauro Lúcio; Venturini, Gabriela Rezende De Oliveira; Castro, Juliana Brandão Pinto De; Ferreira, Maria Elisa Caputo. Repercussões da cirurgia bariátrica na qualidade de vida de pacientes com obesidade: uma

revisão integrativa. *Revista Brasileira De Obesidade, Nutrição E Emagrecimento*, v.12, p.47 - 58, 2018. [Repercussions of bariatric surgery on the quality of life of patients with obesity: an integrative review. *Brazilian Journal Of Obesity, Nutrition And Weight Loss*]

35) Oliveira, L. S. F.; Mazini Filho, M. L.; Castro, J. B. P.; Touguinha, H. M.; Silva, P. C. R.; Ferreira, M. E. C. Repercussões da cirurgia bariátrica na qualidade de vida, no perfil bioquímico e na pressão arterial de pacientes com obesidade mórbida. *Fisioterapia E Pesquisa*, v.25, p.284 - 293, 2018. [Effects of bariatric surgery on quality of life, biochemical profile and blood pressure in patients with morbid obesity. *Physiotherapy And Research*]

Book chapters:

1) Oliveira, L. H. S.; Castro, J. B. P.; Mattos, R. S.; Vale, R. G. S. Prescrição do treinamento de flexibilidade para pessoas com fibromialgia In: *Dor Crônica E Fibromialgia: uma visão interdisciplinar.* Curitiba: CRV, 2019, v.1, p. 215-224.

2) Castro, J. B. P.; Chame, F.; Aguiar, R. S.; Vale, R. G. S. Prescrição dos treinamentos aeróbico e de força para pessoas com fibromialgia In: *Dor Crônica E Fibromialgia: uma visão interdisciplinar.* Curitiba: CRV, 2019, p. 203-214.

Rodrigo Gomes de Souza Vale

Affiliation: Laboratório do Exercício e do Esporte (LABEES), Programa de Pós-Graduação em Ciências do Exercício e do Esporte (PPGCEE), Universidade do Estado do Rio de Janeiro (UERJ) / Universidade Estácio de Sá – campus Cabo Frio, Rio de Janeiro

Education: PhD in Health Sciences (UFRN), Post-Doctorate in Biosciences (UNIRIO)

Research and Professional Experience: Adjunct professor at the Institute of Physical Education and Sports (IEFD) and Post-Graduate Program in Exercise and Sport Sciences, Rio de Janeiro State University, RJ, Brazil (PPGCEE/UERJ). Coordinator of the Exercise and Sport Laboratory (LABEES-UERJ). Full professor, coordinator of the Exercise Physiology Laboratory (LAFIEX) and of the Physical Education course at the Estácio de Sá University (UNESA-Cabo Frio / RJ). Experience in Physical Education and Health: emphasis on Physical Conditioning, Training, Biomechanics, Exercise Physiology, Physical Activity, Health and Quality of Life.

Publications from the Last 3 Years:

Articles in Scientific Journals

1) Matos, Frederico Pecorone; Dantas, Estélio Henrique Martin; De Oliveira, Flávio Boechat; De Castro, Juliana Brandão Pinto; Conceição, Mario Cezar De S Costa; Nunes, Rodolfo De Alkmim Moreira; Vale, Rodrigo Gomes de Souza. Analysis of the pain symptoms, flexibility, and hydroxyproline concentration in individuals with low back pain submitted to Global Postural Re-education and stretching. *Pain Management.*, v.10, p.1 - 177, 2020.
2) Herdy, C. V.; Figueiredo, T.; Silva, G. C.; Galvao, P. V. M.; Vale, R. G. S.; Simão, Roberto. Comparison between anthropometry and multi-frequency bioimpedance for body composition evaluation in Brazilian elite U-20 soccer athletes. *Motricidade (Santa Maria Da Feira),* v.16, p.28 - 38, 2020. [doi:10.6063/motricidade.15557].
3) Silva, Jurandir; Bessi, Fernando; Guimar, Gabriel; Ribeiro, Giovanne; Vale, Rodrigo; Nunes, Rodolfo; Lima, Vicente. Correlação Entre A Medida Antropométrica De Coxa E A Força Em 10 Repetições Máximas. *Inova Saúde,* v.9, p.88 - 99, 2020. [doi:10.18616/inova.v9i2.4544]. [Correlation between the anthropometric measurement of the thigh and the strength at 10 maximum repetitions. *Innovates Health*]

4) Castro, J. B. P.; Lima, Vicente Pinheiro; Santos, A. O. B.; Silva, G. C. P. S. M.; Oliveira, J. G. M.; Silva, J. N. L.; Vale, R. G. S. Correlation analysis between biochemical markers, pain perception, low back functional disability, and muscle strength in postmenopausal women with low back pain. *Journal of Physical Education and Sport,* v.20, p.24 - 30, 2020. [doi:10.7752/jpes.2020.01003].

5) Nodari Junior, R. J.; Vale, R. G. S.; Alberti, A.; Souza, R.; Fin, G.; Dantas, Estélio H. M. Dermatoglyphic traits of Brazilian golfers. *Journal of Physical Education.,* v.31, p.1 - 8, 2020. [doi:10.4025/jphyseduc.v31i1.3103].

6) Gama, D. R. N.; Queiroz, M. A.; Cordeiro, M. C.; Eftimie, J. M.; Vale, R. G. S. Relações entre esportividade e traços de personalidade de esportistas eletrônicos amadores do Rio de Janeiro. *RETOS.,* v.38, p.537 - 542, 2020. [Relationships between sportiness and personality traits of amateur electronic sportsmen in Rio de Janeiro. *RETRO*]

7) Dias Henriques, Ighor Amadeu; Braga De Mello, Danielli; Ribeiro Filho, Kennedy Car; Brandão Pinto De Castro, Juliana; Gomes De Souza Vale, Rodrigo; Rosa, Guilherme. Respuestas de la presión arterial en individuos normotensos sometidos a diferentes intensidades en sesiones de entrenamiento de fuerza. *Revista De Ciencias De La Actividad Física.,* v.21, p.1 - 13, 2020. [doi:10.29035/rcaf.21.1.5]. [Blood pressure responses in normotensive individuals subjected to different intensities in strength training sessions. *Journal of Physical Activity Sciences*]

8) Lima E Silva, L.; Neves, E.; Silva, J.; Alonso, L.; Vale, R.; Nunes, R. The haemodynamic demand and the attributes related to the displacement of the soccer referees in the moments of decision / intervention during the matches. *International Journal of Performance Analysis in Sport,* v.20, p.1 - 12, 2020. [doi:10.1080/24748668.2020.1736937].

9) Castro, Juliana Brandão Pinto De; Brum, Rosana Dias De Oliveira; Pernambuco, Carlos Soares; Vale, Rodrigo Gomes De Souza.

Análise De Correlação Entre Força Muscular, Igf-1 E Autonomia Funcional Em Idosas Com Excesso De Peso Submetidas A Exercícios Resistidos Aquáticos. *Revista de Investigación en Actividades Acuáticas.*, v.3, p.18 - 23, 2019. [doi:10.21134/riaa.v3i5.1575]. [Correlation Analysis Between Muscular Strength, Igf-1 And Functional Autonomy In Overweight Elderly Women Undergoing Aquatic Resistance Exercises. *Revista de Investigación en Acuáticas Activities*]

10) Gama, Dirceu Ribeiro Nogueira Da; Nunes, Rodolfo De Alkmim Moreira; Castro, Juliana Brandão Pinto De; Souza, Camilo Araújo Máximo De; Rodrigues Júnior, Francisco Lopes; Vale, Rodrigo Gomes de Souza. *Analysis of the relationship between personality traits and leadership characteristics of handball coaches of school teams in the state of Rio de Janeiro*, Brazil. Motriz., v.25, p.e101925-, 2019. [doi:10.1590/s1980-6574201900030014].

11) Leite Junior, O. D.; Vale, R. G. S.; Castro, J. B. P.; Oliveira, F. B.; Gama, D. R. N.; Oliveira Filho, G. R.; Fonseca, B. B.; Reis, V. M.; Nunes, R. A. M. Cardiorespiratory responses in maximal cycle ergometry in cardiac rehabilitation. *Journal of Physical Education and Sport.*, v.19, p.393 - 404, 2019.

12) Queiroz, W. R.; Vale, R. G. S.; Silva, L. L. E.; Pernambuco, Carlos Soares; Nunes, R. A. M.; Silva, I. A. S. Comparação dos níveis de agilidade em crianças em idade escolar praticantes e não praticantes de judô: um estudo seccional. *Revista de Educação Física.*, v.88, p.904 - 910, 2019. [Comparison of agility levels in schoolchildren practicing and not practicing judo: a sectional study. *Physical Education Magazine*]

13) Venturini, G. R. O.; Silva, N. S. L.; Almada, L. B.; Castro, J. B. P.; Mazini Filho, M. L.; Vale, R. G. S. Comparação entre indicadores de saúde de alunos do ensino médio das redes federal, estadual e particular de Minas Gerais, Brasil. *Motricidade,* v.15, p.87 - 95, 2019. [doi:10.6063/motricidade.18728].

14) Lima, Bruno Lucas Pinheiro; Leopoldo Junior, Mario Nilton; Santos, Tadeu Leonardo Ribeiro Dos; Silva, Jurandir Baptista Da;

Nunes, Rodolfo De Alkmim Moreira; Vale, Rodrigo Gomes De Souza; Castro, Juliana Brandão Pinto De; Lima, Vicente Pinheiro. Comparación del perfil antropométrico y la aptitud física de los atletas de baloncesto de diferentes posiciones. *Revista De Ciencias De La Actividad Física.*, v.20, p.1 - 13, 2019. [doi:10.29035/rcaf.20.1.6]. [Comparison of the anthropometric profile and physical fitness of basketball athletes of different positions. *Journal of Physical Activity Sciences*]

15) Mello, D. B.; Vale, R. G. S.; Fortes, M. S. R.; Henriques, I.; Sodre, R.; Dias, F. G.; Calassara, T. M.; Selepengue, M. L.; Abreu, G. R. Correlation between nutritional state, blood pressure and waist circumference in sedentary women. *Obesity, Weight Managment & Control.*, v.9, p.152 - 154, 2019. [doi:10.15406/aowmc.2019.09.00291].

16) Corte, J. D.; Rangel, L.; Vale, R. G. S.; Mello, D. B.; Pardo, P. J. M. Does high intensity interval training (HIIT) affect the strength training performance?. *Archivos De Medicina Del Deporte.*, v.36, p.8 - 12, 2019.

17) Nascimento, C. E. R.; Guapyassu, R. M.; Silva, J. B.; Paz, Gabriel Andrade; Gomes, F. D.; Vale, R. G. S.; Nunes, R. A. M.; Lima, Vicente Pinheiro. Efeito subsequente do treinamento de facilitação neuromuscular proprioceptiva nos antagonistas na força dos agonistas em séries múltiplas. *Revista Brasileira De Prescrição E Fisiologia Do Exercício.*, v.13, p.383 - 388, 2019. [Vicente Pinheiro. Subsequent effect of proprioceptive neuromuscular facilitation training on antagonists on the strength of agonists in multiple series. *Brazilian Journal of Prescription and Exercise Physiology*]

18) Santos, B. L. S.; Oliveira, F. B.; Brum, R. D. O.; Vale, R. G. S.; Pernambuco, Carlos Soares. Efeitos da natação no pico expiratório de crianças asmáticas. *Revista de Investigación en Actividades Acuáticas.*, v.3, p.41 - 44, 2019. [doi:10.21134/riaa.v3i6.1576]. [Effects of swimming on the peak expiratory of children with asthma. *Revista de Investigación en Acuáticas Activities*]

19) Marcos-Pardo, Pablo Jorge; Orquin-Castrillón, Francisco Javier; Gea-García, Gemma María; Menayo-Antúnez, Ruperto; González-Gálvez, Noelia; Vale, Rodrigo Gomes De Souza; Martínez-Rodríguez, Alejandro. Effects of a moderate-to-high intensity resistance circuit training on fat mass, functional capacity, muscular strength, and quality of life in elderly: *A randomized controlled trial. Scientific Reports,* v.9, p.7830 - 11, 2019. [doi:10.1038/s41598-019-44329-6].

20) Pernambuco, Carlos Soares; Lima, J. O.; Cortez, A. C. L.; Castro, J. B. P.; Vale, R. G. S.; Oliveira, C. C. C.; Dantas, Estélio H. M. Effects of electroacupuncture on body mass index and quality of life of nurses from Gaffrée and Guinle University Hospital. *International Journal of Development Research.,* v.9, p.25398 - 25402, 2019.

21) Machado, A. F.; Castro, J. B. P.; Bocalini, D. S.; Figueira Junior, A.; Nunes, R. A. M.; Vale, R. G. S. Effects of plyometric training on the performance of 5-km road runners. *Journal of Physical Education and Sport.,* v.2019, p.691 - 695, 2019.

22) Araújo-Gomes, Rafaela Cristina; Valente-Santos, Marcia; Vale, Rodrigo Gomes De Souza; Drigo, Alexandre Janotta; Borba-Pinheiro, Claudio Joaquim. Effects of resistance training, tai chi chuan and mat pilates on multiple health variables in postmenopausal women. *Journal of Human Sport and Exercise,* v.14, p.122 - 139, 2019. [doi:10.14198/jhse.2019.141.10].

23) Silva, L. L. E.; Godoy, E. S.; Neves, E. B.; Vale, R. G. S.; Hall-Lopez, J. A.; Nunes, R. A. M. Frecuencia cardíaca y la distancia recorrida por los árbitros de fútbol durante los partidos: una revisión sistemática. *Archivos De Medicina Del Deporte,* v.36, p.36 - 42, 2019. [Heart rate and distance traveled by soccer referees during matches: a systematic review. *Sports Medicine Archives*]

24) Monteiro-Lago, T.; Cardoso, M. S.; Henriques, I.; Mello, D. B.; Fortes, M. S. R.; Vale, R. G. S.; Rosa, G. Impact of eight weeks of concurrent training on obesity-related biochemical parameters and

cardiometabolic risk factors: a case report. *Obesity, Weight Managment & Control*, v.9, p.98 - 103, 2019.
25) Ramos, A. M.; Alves, J. C. C.; Vale, R. G. S.; Scudese, E.; Senna, Gilmar Weber; Cabral, R. H.; Dantas, Estélio H. M.; Pardono, E. Maximum oxygen intake in hypertensive women submitted to combined training programs with different orders. *Journal of Exercise Physiology Online.*, v.22, p.17 - 25, 2019. Palavras-chave: Exercise, Hypertension, Oxygen intake, VO2max.
26) Gama, D. R. N.; Borges, T. T.; Oliveira, W. J.; Vale, R. G. S. Motivações para o consumo de bens esportivos entre espectadores de esportes eletrônicos. *Lecturas Educación Física Y Deportes.*, v.24, p.66 - 79, 2019.
27) González-Gálvez, Noelia; Poyatos, María Carrasco; Marcos-Pardo, Pablo Jorge; Feito, Yuri; Vale, Rodrigo Gomes De Souza. Pilates Training Induces Changes in the Trunk Musculature of Adolescents. *Revista Brasileira De Medicina Do Esporte (Online)*, v.25, p.235 - 239, 2019. [doi:10.1590/1517-869220192503163535]. [Pilates Training Induces Changes in the Trunk Musculature of Adolescents. *Brazilian Journal of Sports Medicine (Online)*]
28) Nunes, R. A. M.; Silva, J. B.; Machado, A. F.; Menezes, L. S.; Bocalini, D. S.; Silva, I. A. S.; Lima, Vicente Pinheiro; Vale, R. G. S. Prediction of vo2 max in healthy non-athlete men based on ventilatory threshold. *RETOS*, v.35, p.136 - 139, 2019.
29) Castro, J. B. P.; Aguiar, R. S.; Venturini, G. R. O.; Santos, A. O. B.; Silva, G. P.; Lima, T. P.; Principe, V. A.; Vale, R. G. S. The effects of physical exercise on Insulin-Like Growth Factor I in older women: A systematic review. *Journal of Exercise Physiology Online.*, v.22, p.88 - 99, 2019.
30) Castro, J. B. P.; Vale, R. G. S.; Chame, Flávio; Benittez, H. S. P. A.; Silva, J. B.; Nunes, R. A. M.; Mattos, R. S. Análise de conhecimentos e hábitos de hidratação de corredores de rua no município do Rio de Janeiro. *Revista Brasileira De Prescrição E Fisiologia Do Exercício.*, v.12, p.339 - 348, 2018. [Analysis of knowledge and hydration habits of street runners in the city of Rio

de Janeiro. *Brazilian Journal of Prescription and Exercise Physiology*]

31) Oliveira, F. B.; Conceicao, W. C.; Barreto, R.; Carvalho, I. L. S.; Ribeiro, G. M. L.; Vale, R. G. S. Análise de lesões musculoesqueléticas em praticantes de musculação e corrida. *RETOS*, v. 34, p.142 - 145, 2018. [Analysis of musculoskeletal injuries in bodybuilding and running practitioners.]

32) Venturini, Gabriela Rezende De Oliveira; Filho, Mauro Lúcio Mazini; Touguinha, Henrique Menezes; Castro, Juliana Brandão Pinto De; Pereira, Marcos Rodrigues; Vale, Rodrigo Gomes de Souza. Análise do conceito de saúde abordado nas aulas de Educação Física escolar: uma revisão integrativa. *Revista Interdisciplinar de Promoção da Saúde.*, v.1, p.119 - 126, 2018. [doi:10.17058/rips.v1i2.12105]. [Analysis of the health concept covered in school Physical Education classes: an integrative review. Interdisciplinary Journal of Health Promotion]

33) Vale, R. G. S.; Castro, J. B. P.; Mattos, R. S.; Rodrigues, V. F.; Oliveira, F. B.; Rosa, G.; Gama, D. R. N.; Nunes, R. A. M. Analysis of balance, muscle strength, functional autonomy, and quality of life in elderly women submitted to a strength and walking program. *Journal of Exercise Physiology Online.*, v.21, p.13 - 24, 2018.

34) Silva, J. B.; Lima, Vicente Pinheiro; Castro, J. B. P.; Paz, G.; Novaes, Jefferson Da Silva; Nunes, R. A. M.; Vale, R. G. S. Analysis of myoelectric activity, blood lactate concentration and time under tension in repetitions maximum in the squat exercise. *Journal of Physical Education and Sport.*, v.2018, p.2478 - 2485, 2018.

35) Gama, D. R. N.; Nunes, R. A. M.; Guimaraes, G. L.; Silva, L. L. E.; Castro, J. B. P.; Vale, R. G. S. Analysis of the burnout levels of soccer referees working at amateur and professional leagues of Rio de Janeiro, Brazil. *Journal of Physical Education and Sport,* v.18, p.1168 - 1174, 2018.

36) Jati, S. R.; Borba-Pinheiro, Claudio Joaquim; Vale, R. G. S.; Batista, A. J.; Pernambuco, Carlos Soares; Souza, M. J. M.; Moura, A. S.;

Mota, D. L. V.; Figueiredo, D. L.; Dantas, Estélio H. M. Bone density and functional autonomy in post-menopausal women submitted to adapted capoeira exercises and walking. *Journal of Exercise Physiology Online,* v.21, p.214 - 226, 2018.

37) Salarolli, L. C. W.; Barros, R. M. B.; Silva, J. B.; Carvalho, I. L. S.; Vale, R. G. S.; Nunes, R. A. M.; Castro, J. B. P.; Lima, Vicente Pinheiro. Comparison of time under tension, repetition maximum and electromyographic activity in bench press exercise in different speeds execution. *Gazzetta Medica Italiana Archivio Per Le Scienze Mediche,* v.177, p.637 - 644, 2018. [doi:10.23736/s0393-3660.17.03604-x].

38) Alberti, A.; Fin, G.; Vale, R. G. S.; Soares, B. H.; Nodari Junior, R. J. Dermatoglifia: as impressões digitais como marca característica dos atletas de futsal feminino de alto rendimento do Brasil. *Revista Brasileira De Futsal E Futebol.,* v.10, p.193 - 201, 2018. [Dermatoglyphics: fingerprints as a hallmark of high-performance female futsal athletes in Brazil. Brazilian Magazine of Futsal and Football]

39) Borges, Eliane Gomes Da Silva; Vale, Rodrigo Gomes De Souza; Pernambuco, Carlos Soares; Cader, Samaria Ali; Sá, Selma Pedra Chaves; Pinto, Francisco Miguel; Regazzi, Isabel Cristina Ribeiro; Knupp, Virginia Maria De Azevedo Oliveira; Dantas, Estélio Henrique Martin. Effects of dance on the postural balance, cognition and functional autonomy of older adults. *Revista Brasileira De Enfermagem.,* v.71, p.2302 - 2309, 2018. [doi:10.1590/0034-7167-2017-0253].

40) Hall-Lopez, J. A.; Ochoa-Martinez, P. Y.; Monzon, C. O. L.; Vale, R. G. S. Effects of four months of periodized aquatic exercise program on functional autonomy in post-menopausal women with parkinson's disease. *RETOS,* v.33, p.217 - 220, 2018.

41) Vale, R. G. S.; Gama, D. R. N.; Oliveira, F. B.; Almeida, D. S. M.; Castro, J. B. P.; Meza, E. I. A.; Mattos, R. S.; Nunes, R. A. M. Effects of resistance training and chess playing on the quality of life and cognitive performance of elderly women: a randomized

controlled trial. *Journal of Physical Education and Sport.*, v.18, p.1469 - 1477, 2018.

42) Robalinho, M. J. A.; Silva, L. L. E.; Neves, E. B.; Vale, R. G. S.; Nunes, R. A. M. Esporte universitário: percepção de atletas sobre os modelos brasileiro e canadense. *Revista de Educação Física.*, v.87, p.360 - 370, 2018. [University sports: athletes' perception of the Brazilian and Canadian models. *Physical Education Magazine*]

43) Raymundo, Ana Carolina Gago; Pernambuco, Carlos Soares; De Oliveira Brum, Rosana Dias; Castro, Juliana Brandão Pinto De; De Oliveira, Flávio Boechat; Da Gama, Dirceu Ribeiro Nogueira; De Alkmim Moreira Nunes, Rodolfo; De Souza Vale, Rodrigo Gomes. Evaluation of strength, agility and aerobic capacity in Brazilian football players. *Biomedical Human Kinetics.*, v.10, p.25 - 30, 2018. [doi:10.1515/bhk-2018-0005].

44) Dantas, Estélio H. M.; Scudese, E.; Vale, R. G. S.; Senna, Gilmar Weber; Albuquerque, A. P.; Mafra, O.; Scartoni, F. R.; Conceicao, M. C. S. C. Flexibility adaptations in golf players during a whole season. *Journal of Exercise Physiology Online.*, v.21, p.193 - 201, 2018.

45) Lima, Vicente Pinheiro; De Alkmim Moreira Nunes, Rodolfo; Da Silva, Jurandir Baptista; Paz, Gabriel Andrade; Jesus, Marco; De Castro, Juliana Brandão Pinto; Dantas, Estélio Henrique Martin; De Souza Vale, Rodrigo Gomes. Pain perception and low back pain functional disability after a 10-week core and mobility training program: A pilot study. *Journal of Back and Musculoskeletal Rehabilitation.*, v.31, p.1 - 7, 2018. [doi:10.3233/bmr-169739].

46) Silva, I. A. S.; Tavares, A. B. W.; Farias, M. L. F.; Vaisman, M.; Vale, R. G. S.; Conceicao, F. L.; Nunes, R. A. M. Physical activity level, muscle strength, serum levels of IGF-1 and components of the frailty syndrome in the elderly. *Journal of Exercise Physiology Online.*, v.21, p.182 - 192, 2018.

47) Gama, D. R. N.; Barreto, H. D.; Castro, J. B. P.; Nunes, R. A. M.; Vale, R. G. S. Relationships between personality traits and resilience levels of jiu-jitsu and kickboxing Brazilian athletes.

Archives of Budo Science of Martial Arts and Extreme Sports., v.14, p.125 - 133, 2018.

48) Pinto, Jorge Luiz Clemente; Ambrósio, Michelle; Pinheiro Lima, Vicente; Carvalho, Igor Leandro Da Silva; Moreira Nunes, Rodolfo De Alkimim; Vale, Rodrigo Gomes de Souza. Repeticiones máximas y tiempo de tensión entre los ordenes multiarticular para monoarticular y monoarticular para multiarticular en ejercicios resistidos. *Revista De Ciencias De La Actividad Física.*, v.19, p.1 - 11, 2018. [doi:10.29035/rcaf.19.2.6]. [Maximum repetitions and tension time between the orders multiarticular for monoarticular and monoarticular for multiarticular in resisted exercises. *Journal of Physical Activity Sciences*]

49) Fonseca, Renato Tavares; Moreira Nunes, Rodolfo De Alkmim; Pinto De Castro, Juliana Brandão; Lima, Vicente Pinheiro; Silva, Sérgio Gregorio; Dantas, Estélio Henrique Martin; De Souza Vale, Rodrigo Gomes. Aquatic and land plyometric training on the vertical jump and delayed onset muscle soreness in Brazilian soccer players. *Human Movement.*, v.18, p.63 - 70, 2017. [doi:10.1515/humo-2017-0041].

50) Santos, D. F.; Diniz, M. L.; Cardoso, G. A.; Mello, D. B.; Vale, R. G. S.; Dantas, Estélio H. M. Autonomia funcional de idosas fisicamente ativas e insuficientemente ativas de uma cidade do centro sul cearense: um estudo seccional. *Revista de Educação Física.*, v.86, p.250 - 255, 2017. [Functional autonomy of physically active and insufficiently active elderly women in a city in the south of Ceará: a sectional study. *Physical Education Magazine*]

51) Machado, A. F.; Nunes, R. A. M.; Vale, R. G. S.; Figueira Junior, A.; Bocalini, D. S. Body weight based in high intensity interval training: the new calisthenics?. *Revista Terapia Manual.*, v.15, p.1 - 5, 2017.

52) Manceira, B. A. M.; Silva, L. S.; Castro, J. B. P.; Vale, R. G. S.; Nunes, R. A. M.; Lima, Vicente Pinheiro. Comparação do VO2máx e potência anaeróbica de atletas de futebol de base em diferentes posições e categorias. *Revista Brasileira De Futebol.*, v.10, p.35 -

46, 2017. [Comparison of VO2max and anaerobic power of grassroots soccer players in different positions and categories. *Brazilian Football Magazine*]

53) Siqueira, M.; Dantas, G.; Silva, J. B.; Silva, Y. R. L.; Casseres, S. M.; Silva, W. R.; Vale, R. G. S.; Nunes, R. A. M.; Lima, Vicente Pinheiro. Efeito da pré ativação dos antagonistas sobre a atividade eletromiográfica dos agonistas no exercício supino horizontal. *Revista Brasileira De Prescrição E Fisiologia Do Exercício.*, v.11, p.574 - 581, 2017. [Effect of pre-activation of antagonists on the electromyographic activity of agonists in the horizontal bench press exercise. *Brazilian Journal of Prescription and Exercise Physiology*]

54) Oliveira, Leonardo Hernandes De Souza; Mattos, Rafael Da Silva; Castro, Juliana Brandão Pinto De; Barbosa, José Silvio De Oliveira; Chame, Flávio; Vale, Rodrigo Gomes de Souza. Effect of supervised physical exercise on flexibility of fibromyalgia patients. *Revista Dor.*, v.18, p.145 - 149, 2017. [doi:10.5935/1806-0013.20170029].

55) Vale, R. G. S.; Castro, J. B. P.; Oliveira, R. D.; Pernambuco, Carlos Soares; Oliveira, F. B.; Mattos, R. S.; Gama, D. R. N.; Nunes, Rodolfo A. M.; Dantas, Estélio H. M. Effects of hydrogymnastics on IGF-1 and functional autonomy in elderly women. *MOJ Gerontology & Geriatrics.*, v.1, p.1 - 6, 2017.

56) Nunes, Rodolfo De Alkmim Moreira; Castro, Juliana Brandão Pinto De; Silva, Leandro De Lima E; Silva, Jurandir Baptista Da; Godoy, Erik Salum De; Lima, Vicente Pinheiro; Venturini, Gabriela Rezende De Oliveira; Oliveira, Flávio Boechat De; Vale, Rodrigo Gomes de Souza. Estimation of specific VO2max for elderly in cycle ergometer. *Journal of Human Sport and Exercise*, v.12, p.1199 - 1207, 2017. [doi:10.14198/jhse.2017.124.06].

57) Alonso, L.; Silva, L. L. E.; Paulucio, D.; Pompeu, F. A. M. S.; Bezerra, L. O.; Lima, V.; Vale, R. G. S.; Oliveira, M.; Silva Dantas, P. M.; Silva, J. B.; Nunes, R. A. M. Field Tests vs. Post Game GPS

Data in Young Soccer Player Team. *Journal of Exercise Physiology Online.*, v.20, p.102 - 110, 2017.

58) Berbet, C.; Vale, R. G. S.; Silva, L. L. E.; Nunes, R. A. M.; Monteiro, J. C.; Abreu, G. R. Força explosiva em atletas de futebol de campo: uma análise descritiva de acordo com o posicionamento em campo de jogo. *Revista Brasileira De Futebol.*, v.10, p.47 - 57, 2017. [Explosive strength in field soccer athletes: a descriptive analysis according to the position on the playing field. *Brazilian Football Magazine*]

59) Silva, J. B.; Salerno, R.; Passos, V. H.; Paz, G.; Maia, M.; Santanna, H.; Vale, R. G. S.; Nunes, R. A. M.; Lima, Vicente Pinheiro. Hemodynamic subsequent responses between Muay Thai and wrestling professional Brazilian athletes after a high intensity round. *Archives of Budo Science of Martial Arts and Extreme Sports,* v.13, p.41 - 47, 2017.

60) Carvalho, H. S.; Goncalves, F. S.; Vale, R. G. S.; Brito, V. S.; Souza, E. Identificação do uso problemático de jogos eletrônicos em estudantes em uma escola do Rio de Janeiro, Brasil. *Journal of Health Connections.*, v.1, p.19 - 32, 2017.

61) Oliveira, F. B.; Pereira, M. D. M.; Nunes, A. M.; Barreto, R.; Matos, F. P.; Vale, R. G. S. Incidencia de lesiones en la práctica deportiva del motocross. *Revista De Ciencias De La Actividad Física.*, v.18, p.1 - 9, 2017. [Incidence of injuries in motocross sports practice. *Journal of Physical Activity Sciences*]

62) Santana, E. S.; Vale, R. G. S. Índice de desenvolvimento da educação básica na Região dos Lagos, RJ: uma análise dos últimos resultados. *Revista Transdisciplinar Logos E Veritas.*, v.4, p.79 - 90, 2017. [Basic education development index in the Region of Lagos, RJ: an analysis of the latest results. *Transdisciplinary Journal Logos E Veritas*]

63) Castro, J. B. P.; Vale, R. G. S. Insulin-like growth factor I (IGF-1) in older adults: a review. *MOJ Gerontology & Geriatrics.*, v.1, p.1 - 2, 2017.

64) Oliveira, G. R.; Vale, R. G. S.; Oliveira, F. B.; Dias Junior, O. L.; Doria, C.; Nunes, R. A. M. Introduzindo a história da fisioterapia na evolução do futebol brasileiro e europeu. *Fisioterapia Brasil.*, v.18, p.260 - 266, 2017. [Introducing the history of physiotherapy in the evolution of Brazilian and European football. *Physiotherapy Brazil*]

65) Vale, Rodrigo Gomes de Souza; Ferrão, Max Luciano Dias; Nunes, Rodolfo De Alkmim Moreira; Silva, Jurandir Baptista Da; Nodari Júnior, Rudy José; Dantas, Estélio Henrique Martin. *Muscle Strength, GH and IGF-1 in Older Women Submitted to Land and Aquatic Resistance Training.* [doi:10.1590/1517-8692201723 04163788].

66) Herdy, C.; Vale, R. G. S.; Silva, J. B.; Simão, Roberto; Novaes, Jefferson Da Silva; Lima, Vicente Pinheiro; Goncalves, D.; Godoy, E. S.; Selfe, J.; Nunes, R. A. M. Occurrence and type of sports injuries in elite young Brazilian soccer players. *Archivos De Medicina Del Deporte,* v.34, p.140 - 144, 2017.

67) Castro, J. B. P.; Vale, R. G. S.; Aguiar, R. S.; Mattos, R. S. Perfil do estilo de vida de universitários de Educação Física da cidade do Rio de Janeiro. *Revista Brasileira De Ciência E Movimento,* v.25, p.73 - 83, 2017. [Lifestyle profile of Physical Education students in the city of Rio de Janeiro. *Brazilian Journal of Science and Movement*]

68) Costa, R. Q. B.; Silva, L. L. E.; Pimentel, C. E.; Godoy, Erik S.; Gama, D. R. N.; Vale, R. G. S.; Nunes, R. A. M. Perfil sociodemográfico de árbitros de futebol recém-formados no Rio de Janeiro. *Revista de Educação Física.,* v.86, p.284 - 290, 2017. [Sociodemographic profile of recently graduated soccer referees in Rio de Janeiro. *Physical Education Magazine*]

69) Silva, L. L. E.; Paulucio, D.; Pompeu, F. A. M. S.; Alonso, L.; Godoy, E. S.; Bezerra, L. O.; Lima, V.; Vale, R. G. S.; Nunes, R. A. M. Potência anaeróbica e distâncias percorridas durante jogos em jovens atletas de futebol nas categorias Sub-15 e Sub-17. *Revista de Educação Física.*, v.86, p.1 - 7, 2017. [Anaerobic power and distances covered during games for young soccer players in the U-15 and U-17 categories. *Physical Education Magazine*]

70) Lima, Ana Carolina Do Nascimento; Oliveira, Flavio Boechat De; Avolio, Gabriela Pereira; Silva, Giselly Dias Da; Silva, Paula Soares Da; Vale, Rodrigo Gomes de Souza. Prevalence of low back pain and interference with quality of life of pregnant women. *Revista Dor,* v.18, p.119 - 123, 2017. [doi:10.5935/1806-0013.20170024].
71) Lima, Vicente Pinheiro; Nunes, R. A. M.; Ribeiro, C. C.; Alves, L. R.; Carvalho, I. L. S.; Vale, R. G. S. Prevalência de lesões em praticantes de Jiu-Jitsu: um estudo descritivo. *Revista de Educação Física.,* v.86, p.31 - 37, 2017. [Injury prevalence in Jiu-Jitsu practitioners: a descriptive study. *Physical Education Magazine*]
72) Silva, J. B.; Lima, Vicente Pinheiro; Novaes, Jefferson Da Silva; Castro, J. B. P.; Nunes, R. A. M.; Vale, R. G. S. Time under tension, muscular activation, and blood lactate responses to perform 8, 10, and 12RM in the bench press exercise. *Journal of Exercise Physiology Online.,* v.20, p.41 - 54, 2017.
73) Lima, Vicente Pinheiro; Nunes, R. A. M.; Castro, J. B. P.; Souza, C. C.; Rodrigues, F. A. B.; Vale, R. G. S. Variações hemodinâmicas em idosas pré e pós-exercícios em hidroginástica. *Revista de Educação Física.,* v.86, p.18 - 24, 2017. [Hemodynamic variations in elderly women before and after exercise in water aerobics. *Physical Education Magazine.*]

Books:

1) Vale, R. G. S.; Santana, E. S. Atividade física e envelhecimento. Rio de Janeiro: *SESES,* 2019, v.1. p. 121. ISBN: 9788555487224. [Physical activity and aging.]
2) Vale, R. G. S.; Pernambuco, Carlos Soares; Alias, A.; Dantas, Estélio H. M. *Bases de entrenamiento deportivo para adultos mayores: procedimientos de evaluación.* Madrid, Espanha: Dykinson, S. L., 2018, v.1. p. 201. ISBN: 9788491489641. [*Bases of sports training for older adults: evaluation procedures*]

Book chapters:

1) Mello, D. B.; Dantas, G. H. M.; Vale, R. G. S. Fisiologia do exercício aplicada ao ciclismo indoor In: *Ciclismo indoor: bases científicas e metodológicas.* 2 ed.São Paulo: RV Editorial, 2020, v.1, p. 41-74. ISBN: 9786587118000. [Exercise physiology applied to indoor cycling In: *Indoor cycling: scientific and methodological bases.*]
2) Borba-Pinheiro, Claudio Joaquim; Albuquerque, A. P.; Vale, R. G. S.; Carvalho, M. C. G. A.; Jesus, F. P.; Silva, A. M. B. F.; Figueiredo, N. M. A.; Santos, C. A. S.; Dantas, E. H. M.; Costa, L. F. G. R. Treinamento neuromuscular na prevenção e controle das quedas em idosos In: *Prevenção de quedas em idosos.* 1 ed. Madrid, Espanha: Editorial Dykinson, 2020, v.1, p. 101-128. ISBN: 9788413247670. [Neuromuscular training in the prevention and control of falls in the elderly In: *Prevention of falls in the elderly*]
3) Salomao, P. T.; Vale, R. G. S.; Conceicao, M. C. S. C.; Dantas, Estélio H. M. Avaliação subjetiva In: *Manual de avaliação da flexibilidade.* 1 ed. São Paulo: Manole, 2019, v.1, p. 107-114. ISBN: 9788520458501 [Subjective evaluation In: *Flexibility assessment manual*]
4) Vale, R. G. S.; Barreto, Ana Cristina Lopes Y Glória; Conceicao, M. C. S. C.; Dantas, Estélio H. M. Fundamentos estatísticos aplicados à avaliação da flexibilidade In: *Manual de avaliação da flexibilidade.* 1 ed. São Paulo: Manole, 2019, v.1, p. 191-208. ISBN: 9788520458501 [Statistical fundamentals applied to the flexibility assessment In: *Flexibility assessment manual.*]
5) Oliveira, Leonardo Hernandes De Souza; Castro, J. B. P.; Mattos, R. S.; Vale, R. G. S. Prescrição do treinamento de flexibilidade para pessoas com fibromialgia In: *Dor crônica e fibromialgia: uma visão interdisciplinar.* 1 ed. Curitiba: CRV, 2019, v.1, p. 215-224. ISBN: 9788544432853. [Prescription of flexibility training for people with fibromyalgia In: *Chronic pain and fibromyalgia: an interdisciplinary view*]

6) Castro, J. B. P.; Chame, Flávio; Aguiar, R. S.; Vale, R. G. S. Prescrição dos treinamentos aeróbico e de força para pessoas com fibromialgia In: *Dor crônica e fibromialgia: uma visão interdisciplinar.* 1 ed. Curitiba: CRV, 2019, v.1, p. 203-214. ISBN: 9788544432853. [Prescription of aerobic and strength training for people with fibromyalgia In: *Chronic pain and fibromyalgia: an interdisciplinary view*]

7) Silva, F. B.; Pernambuco, Carlos Soares; Brum, R. D. O.; Santana, E. S.; Pinto, S. M.; Vale, R. G. S. Análise da glicemia capilar em idosos submetidos a três diferentes protocolos de exercício físico In: *Métodos inovadores de exercícios físicos na saúde: prescrição baseada em evidências.* 1 ed. São Paulo: Conselho Regional de Educação Física da 4ª Região, 2018, v.1, p. 135-143. ISBN: 9788594418265. [Analysis of capillary glycemia in the elderly undergoing three different physical exercise protocols In: *Innovative methods of physical exercise in health: evidence-based prescription*]

8) Almeida, L. B.; Pernambuco, Carlos Soares; De Oliveira Brum, Rosana Dias; Santana, E. S.; Pinto, S. M.; Dublasievicz, R. M.; Vale, R. G. S. Domínios cognitivos em idosos submetidos a um programa de exercícios resistidos In: *Métodos inovadores de exercícios físicos na saúde: prescrição baseada em evidências.* 1 ed. São Paulo: Conselho Regional de Educação Física da 4ª Região, 2018, v.1, p. 59-68. ISBN: 9788594418265. [Cognitive domains in the elderly undergoing a resistance exercise program In: *Innovative methods of physical exercise in health: evidence-based prescription.*]

9) Amaral, K. N. O.; Torres, E. M. S.; Vale, R. G. S.; Figueiredo, D. L.; Borba-Pinheiro, Claudio Joaquim. Efeito hipotensor agudo em mulheres de idade avançada após diferentes ordens de exercícios resistidos In: *Métodos inovadores de exercícios físicos na saúde: prescrição baseada em evidências.* 1 ed. São Paulo: Conselho Regional de Educação Física da 4ª Região – São Paulo, 2018, v.1, p. 43-57. ISBN: 9788594418265. [Acute hypotensive effect in older

women after different orders of resistance exercise In: *Innovative methods of physical exercise in health: evidence-based prescription*]

10) Vale, R. G. S.; Silva, R. V. V.; Figueira, Helena A.; Correa, D. G.; Gomes, A. R. S.; Silva, Rosilane Barros da. Flexibilidade e a maturidade In: *Alongamento e flexionamento*. 6 ed. Barueri, SP: Manole, 2018, v.1, p. 208-241. ISBN: 9788520454473. [Flexibility and maturity In: *Stretching and flexing*]

11) Lopes Junior, D. B.; Mendes, R. A. B.; Melo, G. E. L.; Saraiva, A. R.; Vale, R. G. S.; Borba-Pinheiro, Claudio Joaquim. Treinamento resistido linear ou funcional, qual método de exercício é o mais eficaz para a força muscular e autonomia funcional de mulheres em idade avançada? In: *Métodos inovadores de exercícios físicos na saúde: prescrição baseada em evidências*. 1 ed. São Paulo: Conselho Regional de Educação Física da 4ª Região, 2018, v.1, p. 119-134. ISBN: 9788594418265. [Linear or functional resistance training, which exercise method is the most effective for muscle strength and functional autonomy in older women? In: *Innovative methods of physical exercise in health: evidence-based prescription*.]

12) Borba-Pinheiro, Claudio Joaquim; Albuquerque, A. P.; Vale, R. G. S.; Carvalho, M. C. G. A.; Jesus, F. P.; Silva, A. M. B. F.; Figueiredo, Nébia Maria Almeida De. A prática de exercícios físicos como forma de prevenção In: *Aspectos biopsicossociais do envelhecimento e a prevenção de quedas na terceira idade*. 1 ed. Joaçaba, SC: Editora Unoesc, 2017, v.1, p. 171-232. ISBN: 9788584221455. [The practice of physical exercises as a form of prevention In: *Biopsychosocial aspects of aging and the prevention of falls in old age*]

13) Vale, R. G. S.; Silva, J. B.; Aguiar, R. S.; Castro, J. B. P.; Borba-Pinheiro, Claudio Joaquim. Exame físico no idoso In: *Aspectos biopsicossociais do envelhecimento e a prevenção de quedas na terceira idade*. 1 ed. Joaçaba, SC: Editora Unoesc, 2017, v.1, p. 71-112. ISBN: 9788584221455. [Physical examination in the elderly In: *Biopsychosocial aspects of aging and the prevention of falls in old age.*]

INDEX

A

active transport, 12, 18
activity level, 7, 11, 128
adaptations, 9, 25, 26, 53, 73, 75, 76, 90, 93, 128
adolescents, 2, 10, 11, 12, 13, 16, 17, 18, 19, 23, 24, 25, 26, 27, 28, 30, 31, 32
adult obesity, 3
adulthood, 4, 11, 13, 14, 29, 30, 31
adults, 2, 7, 11, 13, 19, 22, 27, 33, 36, 56, 57, 59, 60, 62, 127, 131
aerobic capacity, 54, 117, 128
aerobic exercise, 10, 87, 88
age, 11, 13, 14, 24, 36, 37, 38, 39, 40, 41, 42, 44, 45, 47, 48, 51, 82
aging, iv, v, vii, viii, 35, 36, 37, 38, 39, 40, 42, 43, 44, 45, 46, 47, 48, 49, 50, 51, 52, 53, 54, 55, 56, 57, 58, 59, 60, 61, 62, 78, 82, 91, 93, 112, 133, 136, 137
aging process, 37, 38, 39, 40, 42, 43, 46, 48, 52, 53
alpha-tocopherol, 92

angiogenesis, 75, 82, 97
anthropometric modifications, 40
antioxidant, viii, 72, 74, 76, 78, 79, 83, 84, 85, 88, 89, 91, 92, 93, 96
antioxidant defense system, viii, 72, 83, 84
athletes, 84, 92, 115, 118, 120, 128, 131
atrophy, 44, 45, 47, 87
autonomy, viii, 36, 38, 39, 55, 116, 126, 127, 130

B

back pain, 66, 100, 106, 113, 118, 120, 121, 128, 133
balance training, viii, 36, 53, 54
baroreceptor, 43
basic needs, 37
beneficial effect, 15
benefits, 10, 11, 15, 21, 22, 30, 50, 55, 60
biochemistry, 72, 92, 95, 96
biomarkers, 86
biomolecules, 78

blood, viii, 42, 43, 45, 72, 75, 87, 116, 123, 126, 133
blood plasma, 75
blood pressure, 43, 45, 123
blood vessels, 42, 43
body composition, 5, 6, 7, 10, 14, 28, 30, 41, 49, 59, 60, 88, 120
body fat, 5, 7, 9, 23, 41, 42, 68, 69, 103, 104
body fluid, 75
body mass index, 42, 115, 124
body shape, 41
body weight, iv, v, vii, 1, 2, 3, 4, 6, 7, 8, 9, 10, 13, 14, 15, 16, 17, 21, 23, 25, 26, 27, 29, 33, 41, 42, 50, 51, 129
Brazil, 20, 35, 37, 42, 63, 67, 69, 71, 98, 102, 104, 105, 106, 111, 114, 117, 120, 122, 126
breakdown, 79, 80
breathing, 44, 80, 81
by-products, 80, 81

C

calcium, 47, 76, 78, 81, 88, 90
caloric intake, 5, 26
caloric restriction, 5, 25
cancer, 2, 41, 48
carbon dioxide, 54, 73
cardiac output, 43
cardiorespiratory or aerobic training, viii, 36
cardiovascular disease, 32, 41, 42, 58
cardiovascular function, 43
cardiovascular system, 42, 54, 57
cell signaling, 83
cellular immunity, 47
central nervous system, 15, 44, 53
cerebral palsy, 66, 101
cerebrovascular disease, 48
chain propagation, 84
childhood, viii, 2, 3, 4, 11, 13, 14, 17, 22, 24, 26, 29, 30, 31, 32, 40

children, 3, 4, 10, 11, 12, 13, 14, 16, 17, 18, 19, 20, 21, 22, 24, 25, 26, 27, 28, 29, 30, 31, 32, 33, 36, 39, 65, 100
cognitive performance, 117, 127
concept of physical fitness, viii, 36
connective tissue, 46, 52
consumption, ix, 3, 5, 44, 94
controlled trials, 26, 27, 32
coordination, 20, 26, 29, 49
coronary artery disease, 47

D

daily living, vii, 1, 39, 46, 50
defense mechanisms, 9, 83, 84
definition of oxidative stress and reactive oxygen species (ROS), viii, 72, 73, 74, 75, 76, 77, 78, 79, 80, 81, 82, 83, 84, 85, 88, 94, 95
depression, 2, 39, 42, 48
depressive symptoms, 3
developed countries, 7, 36, 39
diabetes, 38, 41, 47
diaphragm, 97, 98
diet, 38, 84, 93, 96
dietary intake, 4, 5, 6, 20
disability, 2, 37, 51, 113, 118, 121, 128
diseases, 2, 37, 38, 39, 42, 47, 48, 50, 92
displacement, 64, 98, 121
distribution, 12, 41, 42, 68, 69, 103, 104
dose-response relationship, 62

E

education, 11, 16, 113, 120
effects of high-intensity resistance training in skeletal muscle, viii, 72
elderly, iv, v, vii, viii, 35, 36, 37, 38, 39, 40, 42, 43, 44, 45, 46, 47, 48, 49, 50, 51, 52, 53, 54, 55, 57, 58, 60, 61, 62, 64, 99, 109, 112, 114, 116, 117, 118, 122, 124,

126, 127, 128, 129, 130, 133, 134, 135, 137
elderly population, 36, 37
endocrine, viii, 36, 46, 48, 73, 92
endocrine system, viii, 36, 48
endurance, viii, 36, 50, 51, 55, 73, 86, 95, 97
energy, vii, 2, 4, 5, 6, 7, 8, 9, 10, 16, 17, 18, 20, 21, 22, 24, 30, 31, 33, 41, 54, 74, 75, 78
energy balance, viii, 2, 4, 5, 6, 7, 8, 9, 16, 17, 18, 21, 23, 24, 30, 31
energy expenditure, vii, 2, 4, 5, 6, 7, 8, 9, 10, 16, 18, 21, 22
energy flux, vii, 2, 6, 7, 8, 9, 16, 24
energy intake, viii, 2, 4, 5, 6, 8, 16, 20, 30
enlargement, 40
environment, vii, 1, 3, 4, 9, 16, 24, 30, 40
environmental factors, 38
environmental stress, 38
environments, 9, 16, 30
enzymes, 76, 78, 82, 83, 86
evidence, 12, 14, 27, 28, 32, 48, 50, 54, 74, 79, 82
excess body weight, vii, 1, 2, 3, 4, 9, 16, 41
exercise, iv, viii, ix, 2, 4, 5, 7, 10, 14, 17, 18, 19, 21, 23, 24, 25, 26, 27, 30, 31, 32, 33, 43, 44, 48, 49, 50, 51, 53, 55, 56, 57, 58, 60, 62, 65, 67, 72, 73, 74, 75, 76, 77, 81, 84, 85, 86, 87, 88, 89, 90, 91, 92, 93, 94, 95, 96, 97, 100, 102, 106, 108, 110, 111, 112, 115, 116, 117, 120, 123, 124, 125, 126, 127, 128, 130, 131, 133, 134, 135, 136
exercise program, 10, 17, 21, 49, 51, 127
exercises, 5, 15, 31, 43, 44, 49, 50, 51, 52, 53, 54, 55, 66, 72, 77, 84, 101, 108, 117, 127

F

fat, 5, 18, 25, 30, 32, 33, 41, 42, 43, 68, 93, 103, 124
fibers, 45, 46, 73, 75, 76, 77, 85, 95
fitness, vii, viii, 1, 2, 3, 11, 13, 14, 16, 17, 19, 23, 25, 26, 29, 31, 49, 54, 55, 69, 104
flexibility, viii, 36, 49, 50, 52, 53, 107, 113, 117, 120, 130
flexibility training, viii, 36, 52, 107, 117, 134
food, 5, 9, 21, 25, 28, 33, 37
food intake, 25, 33
formation, 43, 77, 82, 87
fractures, 45, 47, 51, 54
free radicals, ix, 72, 74, 83, 84, 89
functional changes, 37, 39, 44

G

gene expression, 77
genes, 4, 30, 77, 89
genetic factors, 40
glucose, 30, 69, 74, 75, 104
glucose tolerance, 30
glutathione, 77, 83
growth factor, 115, 131
growth hormone, 46, 48

H

health, vii, 1, 2, 3, 7, 9, 10, 12, 16, 18, 19, 21, 29, 31, 32, 33, 37, 41, 45, 46, 47, 49, 50, 51, 52, 55, 59, 63, 72, 87, 98, 110, 124
health care, 3
health care costs, 3
health effects, 3
health promotion, 2, 18, 21, 57, 116, 126

human, viii, 2, 7, 9, 16, 27, 28, 53, 57, 74, 85, 90, 92
human body, 27, 74, 85
hydrogen, 78, 85, 88, 89, 93
hydrogen peroxide, 78, 85, 88, 89, 93
hyperinsulinemia, 92
hyperlipidemia, 41
hypertension, 41, 47
hypertrophy, 73, 77

I

immune function, 47
immune system, viii, 36, 40, 47
incidence, 42, 47, 49, 54
independence, viii, 36, 38, 39, 50, 52, 55
individuals, 9, 31, 38, 40, 43, 44, 47, 77, 82, 85, 113, 120
industrial revolution, 37
industrialized countries, 22
injuries, 45, 51, 53, 65, 67, 77, 100, 102, 132
insulin, 32, 81, 88, 97, 115
interference, 133
interpersonal relations, 37
interpersonal relationships, 37
intervention, vii, 2, 4, 11, 12, 15, 16, 18, 20, 21, 23, 27, 28, 30, 31, 64, 99, 121
intervention strategies, vii, 2, 4, 11, 12, 16
intracellular calcium, 78

L

life expectancy, 37
lipid peroxidation, 75, 82, 90, 92
locomotor, 10, 52
longitudinal study, 23

M

maximum oxygen consumption, 43
measurement, 27, 52, 97
meta-analysis, 20, 22, 26, 27, 30, 32, 62
metabolic disorder, 48
metabolic syndrome, 41, 64, 69, 99, 105
military, 66, 68, 69, 70, 101, 103, 105
military tasks, 70, 105
mitochondria, 76, 78, 79, 80, 81, 89
molecules, ix, 72, 75, 78, 82, 83, 84
mortality, 2, 36, 42, 50, 60, 63
motor competence, vii, 1, 2, 3, 4, 10, 13, 14, 15, 16, 17, 18, 19, 21, 29, 32
motor development, 14, 15, 17, 22
motor neurons, 45
motor skills, 3, 23, 29, 65, 100
motor task, 13
muscle atrophy, 42, 74, 76
muscle contraction, 73, 74, 75, 79, 80, 81, 82, 93
muscle mass, 46, 59
muscle performance, 75
muscle strength, viii, ix, 15, 36, 45, 49, 50, 51, 59, 66, 68, 72, 73, 74, 82, 101, 103, 113, 116, 121, 126, 128
muscles, ix, 41, 44, 46, 50, 52, 54, 72, 74, 77, 80, 81
muscular dystrophy, 82
musculoskeletal, viii, 36, 40, 45, 67, 74, 86, 102
musculoskeletal system, viii, 36, 45, 74

N

negative effects, ix, 72, 74
nervous system, viii, 15, 36, 44, 53
neurodegenerative diseases, 46
neurotransmitters, 42, 45
neutrophils, 91, 94
nicotinamide, 79, 94

nitric oxide, 78, 85, 94
nutritional state, 123

O

obesity, vii, 2, 3, 4, 11, 14, 16, 18, 19, 20, 22, 23, 24, 25, 26, 27, 28, 29, 30, 31, 32, 33, 56, 59, 65, 67, 68, 92, 99, 102, 103, 107, 119, 123, 124
obesity prevention, 18, 22, 32
overweight, vii, 2, 11, 14, 15, 16, 19, 20, 23, 24, 27, 29, 30, 32, 33, 56, 114, 122
oxidation, 75, 76, 78, 82, 83, 95
oxidative damage, viii, 72, 77, 78, 90, 91
oxidative stress, iv, v, vii, viii, 71, 72, 73, 74, 76, 77, 79, 82, 84, 85, 86, 87, 89, 90, 91, 92, 93, 94, 95, 96, 97, 111
oxygen, viii, 54, 72, 73, 75, 78, 80, 81, 83, 93, 94, 125
oxygen consumption, ix, 72, 73, 75, 78, 83

P

pain, 47, 113, 120, 121
pain perception, 113, 121
pathological aging, 38
personality traits, 114, 118, 122, 128
phosphate, 74, 78, 80, 94
physial fitness, 13
physical activity, vii, viii, 1, 2, 4, 8, 18, 19, 20, 21, 22, 23, 24, 25, 26, 27, 28, 29, 30, 31, 32, 33, 35, 37, 43, 49, 59
physical education, 12, 30
physical exercise, 43, 48, 50, 53, 54, 55, 67, 73, 74, 83, 92, 94, 96, 102, 115, 125, 130
physical fitness, iv, v, vii, viii, 1, 2, 3, 4, 10, 13, 14, 15, 16, 17, 19, 31, 32, 36, 41, 48, 49, 56, 57, 59, 60, 62, 63, 64, 69, 70, 72, 98, 99, 104, 105, 114, 123
physical inactivity, 2, 3, 23, 25, 46, 50, 59
physical structure, 29

physical training, 36, 83
physiology, iv, v, vii, viii, 7, 9, 35, 36, 37, 40, 58, 59, 60, 62, 85, 86, 87, 88, 89, 90, 91, 92, 93, 94, 95, 96, 97, 98, 105, 106, 111, 112, 115, 116, 117, 120, 123, 125, 126, 127, 128, 130, 131, 133, 134
physiology of aging, iv, vii, viii, 36, 40
pilot study, 118, 128
population, vii, viii, 10, 23, 26, 27, 36, 37, 40, 55, 75
primary school, 19, 21, 23, 29, 30, 32
professionals, 37, 55, 69, 104
protein kinases, 76
protein-protein interactions, 81
proteins, 76, 77, 81, 83, 90
public health, 16, 25, 26, 50, 51

Q

quality of life, 3, 37, 46, 115, 116, 117, 124, 126, 127, 133

R

reactive oxygen, vii, viii, 72, 73, 80, 87, 90, 91, 96, 98
recommendations, iv, 2, 10, 25, 33, 50, 60
referees, 64, 65, 98, 100, 117, 121, 126
resistance, vii, viii, 5, 15, 20, 21, 22, 31, 44, 50, 51, 56, 58, 62, 67, 71, 72, 73, 76, 86, 88, 90, 92, 102, 108, 117, 124, 127
resistance training, iv, vii, viii, 15, 20, 22, 31, 51, 56, 62, 66, 67, 71, 72, 73, 76, 86, 101, 102, 108, 117, 124, 127, 132, 136
respiratory system, viii, 36, 44
response, viii, 2, 9, 21, 43, 45, 73
reticulum, 78, 81, 88, 95
risk, 2, 3, 14, 15, 19, 29, 31, 32, 40, 41, 45, 48, 50, 52, 54, 55, 57, 58, 59, 107, 125
risk factors, 19, 32, 40, 48, 107, 125

S

school, 12, 18, 20, 23, 25, 26, 114, 122
sedentary behavior, vii, 1, 27, 29
sedentary lifestyle, 3, 7, 9, 54
skeletal muscle, vii, viii, 41, 44, 46, 57, 59, 62, 71, 73, 74, 75, 77, 78, 79, 80, 81, 82, 83, 85, 87, 88, 89, 90, 91, 92, 93, 94, 95, 96, 97
skin, 40, 41, 67, 68, 102, 103
soccer, 64, 65, 91, 98, 100, 117, 120, 121, 126, 129, 132
species, vii, viii, 72, 73, 80, 87, 90, 91, 93, 94, 96, 98
stages and types of aging, viii, 36
strength training, 15, 21, 48, 49, 50, 51, 60, 67, 73, 102, 113, 118, 123
strength training/resistance training, 50
stress, viii, 42, 72, 79, 85, 93, 95, 96, 98
supplementation, 92, 95, 96
susceptibility, 47, 90
symptoms, 38, 113, 120

T

temperature, 67, 68, 69, 73, 85, 102, 103, 104
tension, 116, 117, 126, 127, 133
testosterone, 48, 69, 104
therapy, 31, 66, 101
tissue, 42, 45, 52, 73, 75, 78, 87, 92
training, vii, viii, 15, 20, 22, 27, 30, 31, 32, 36, 48, 49, 51, 54, 56, 62, 67, 69, 71, 72, 73, 74, 75, 76, 83, 84, 86, 88, 89, 91, 96, 97, 102, 104, 107, 108, 111, 113, 115, 117, 118, 123, 124, 125, 127, 128, 129
training programs, 125
transcription, 76, 84, 95
transformation, 41, 82, 97
treatment, 31, 66, 100, 106
trial, 28, 29, 117, 124, 128
tumor necrosis factor, 73

V

vascular diseases, 42
ventilation, 44, 91
vestibular system, 53
vitamin C, 88
vitamins, 83, 84

W

walking, viii, 36, 39, 46, 50, 53, 55, 62, 116, 126, 127
water absorption, 40
weight gain, viii, 2, 4, 5, 8, 9, 16, 33
weight loss, 6, 9, 15, 19, 25, 26, 42
weight management, 4, 6, 10, 13, 21, 42
weight status, 19, 20, 23, 24
well-being, 2, 9, 13, 16

Y

young adults, 21, 31, 95
young people, 26, 36
young women, 32